Allure

Other books by Julie Davis

30 Days to a Better Bust
30 Days to a Beautiful Bottom
30 Days to Healthy Hair
How to Get Married
The Sweet Dreams Body Book
20 Minutes a Day to a Healthier Back

Allure

How to Be the Woman Men Want and Women Want to Be

Julie Davis

•

Illustrations by Elaine Yabroudy
Photographs by Peter Zander

BANTAM BOOKS
Toronto • New York • London • Sydney

ALLURE

A Bantam Book / June 1984

Book design by Lurelle Cheverie

Library of Congress Cataloging in Publication Data

Davis, Julie, 1956-
Allure: how to be the woman men want and women want to be

1. Beauty, Personal. 1. Title.
RA778.D247 1984   646.7'2   83-25655
ISBN 0-553-34074-3

Published simultaneously in the United States and Canada

Bantam Books are published by Bantam Books, Inc.
Its trademark, consisting of the words "Bantam Books"
and the portrayal of a rooster, is Registered in the
United States Patent and Trademark Office and in other
countries. Marca Registrada. Bantam Books, Inc.,
666 Fifth Avenue, New York, New York 10103.

PRINTED IN THE UNITED STATES OF AMERICA

FG   0 9 8 7 6 5 4 3 2 1

For Michele, Elaine and Annemarie,
three women who understand the magic of allure

Contents

Acknowledgements   ix
Introduction   1

Week One: Beauty   3
Day 1   : Creating a Beautiful Self-Image   5
Day 2   : Allure of the Eyes   11
Day 3   : Allure of the Lips   25
Day 4   : Allure of the Hands   29
Day 5   : Forgotten Art of Comportment   39
Day 6   : Working with Beauty Flaws   47
Day 7   : Putting Beauty to Work for You   93

Week Two: Style   99
Day 8   : Developing Your Own Style   101
Day 9   : Fashion Forum I: Image Dressing for Daytime   111
Day 10   : Fashion Forum II: Image Dressing for
          Nighttime   119
Day 11   : Impact of Perfume   127
Day 12   : Hairstyle: an Essential Fashion   133
Day 13   : Lifestyle: Easy Surroundings   141
Day 14   : Putting Style to Work for You   147

Week Three: Attitude   153
Day 15   : Attitude: Taking Beauty and Style to the
          Next Dimension   155
Day 16   : Be Interesting   159
Day 17   : Be Interested   169
Day 18   : How to Project at Work   173
Day 19   : How to Project at Play   181
Day 20   : Your Many Faces   189
Day 21   : Putting It All Together   195

ACKNOWLEDGMENTS

Capturing the essence of allure on film is no easy task. Well-deserved praise belongs to all my wonderful "models": Michele Salcedo, Elaine Yabroudy and Annemarie Wurche, three beautiful, talented women; Charles Geffen, the "leading man"; Ron Ahlert, Andrea Salcedo, Belinda Sym-Smith, and Kim Larkin, my brother, for the supporting roles; Robert Sternbach, restauranteur par excellence, who not only posed but also opened his delicious *Tastings* restaurant to us for our glamorous backdrop; Roslyn Targ, my agent, who brought her special allure to this project; and Brad Miner, my terrific editor, who went beyond the call of duty by agreeing to step in front of the camera—his support and assistance made writing this book even more of a treat.

Special thank-you's go to those who made it work from behind the scenes: Carl of Bumble & Bumble, for his hairstyling wizardry; Patrick Swan, for his miraculous makeup transformations; Liz Claiborne whose fashions are all a woman needs to go from a morning jog in the park to an afternoon board meeting to the most gala night on the town; Carol for Eva Graham whose exciting jewelry is always perfect; Linda Grey who graciously offered her executive suite at Bantam as the office locale; Peter Zander who captured the magic through his lens; and Elaine, again, for translating through her artwork those few elements that eluded the camera.

ALLURE:
The Determining
Factor

W hat is it that makes heads turn when a certain woman enters a room? What gets people to listen to her and, more importantly, to respond to her? What is it all the other women in that room wish they had?

Call it sex appeal, charisma, pizzazz, or allure, as I do, it is the key to being the woman who stands out in the crowd, who dazzles every audience. It is the polish and the sparkle that makes everything else you do for yourself work that much better. The best part about it? It comes from within: You can create it.

What is allure? Very simply it is self-confidence, a quality that gives a woman the courage to be provocative and daring, more special than the rest. Why does it seem so hard to attain? Because of fear, that terrifying emotion that keeps you from try- ing, from doing and learning. Confidence is built on experience;

fear stops you from gaining that experience, from expressing opinions and desires, from going after that promotion, even from wearing a certain style of clothing, or walking into a restaurant by yourself and feeling at ease.

To conquer fear, you need to build a strong foundation of self-esteem. To accomplish this, you need to believe in your own worth and to project this belief through a dynamic attitude, a strong sense of personal style, and by presenting a terrific appearance. These three qualities work hand in hand to make you see yourself as the gregarious woman you want to be; one who goes after what she wants, be it a new career or a new man, and who gets it—the woman you've always dreamed of being, but were afraid to become. Truth is, you can be that woman, if you take the chance and make the effort. I'll tell you how—how I did it for myself, how you can do it easily and effectively.

Mine is a comprehensive, three week, step-by-step plan. Each of the 21 days is a building block: you may start with any week you choose and read one "day" at a time, or one "day" every other day, or one a week—your decision. Put them all together and you create a new you.

I've included many photographs to show you how the goal is accomplished. The women featured are not professional models. They are women who learned, just as you will, how to capitalize on their assets to become not only the kind of woman every man wants, but also the woman every woman wants to be.

Beauty

B eauty is overrated. The movie *10* showed us that without the intelligence to back it up, beauty is worth nothing more than a spread in *Playboy*. And yet first impressions are visual ones. And we are, however wrongly, still judged, at least in part, by our appearance—men as often as women. Conclusion: until our values become less superficial, we need to pay attention to our looks. Certainly there is nothing wrong with wanting to look attractive (whether or not you are a woman who readily admits to it), as long as you don't neglect the rest.

This week is designed to help you make the most of your physical appearance; to look your best and then to free you to move on to other pursuits.

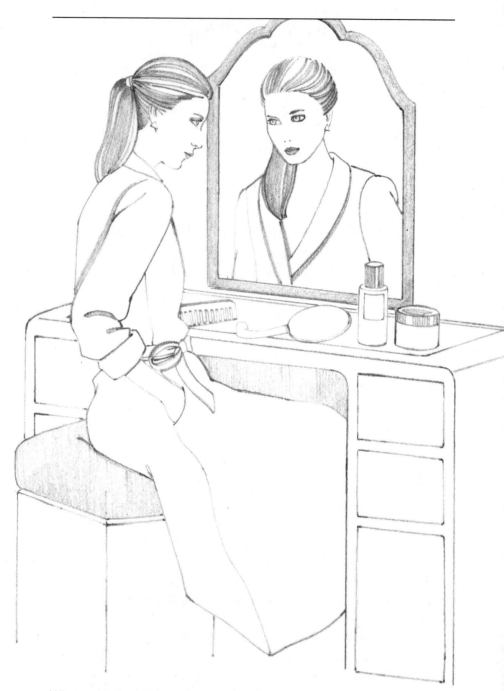

*When you look into the mirror,
see only the potential, never the flaws.*

Creating a Beautiful Self-Image

If I were to sit down and make a list of my physical shortcomings (and I can assure you that I have), I'd put down that my eyes are too close together, that I have no eyebrows to speak of, that I need more "legwork," that . . . Must I go on? You get the picture: look hard enough and you'll find plenty of flaws.

But when the world sees me, it sees only the great look I have made for myself, through makeup, the way I style my hair, my clothes and, even more than all these put together, my attitude. Because when I do look in the mirror, I no longer moan about the flaws that should have been assets. I see only the potential and I make the most of it. When I walk away from that mirror, I have one thought in mind: I am fabulous. And you know what? That's exactly what everyone else perceives.

Projecting Your Potential:
The Mirror Exercise

This little attitude developer is to be practiced every single morning in front of your bathroom mirror. At first, you will undoubtedly feel embarrassed as it involves talking to yourself. Well, that's a feeling you'll quickly overcome. If you are worried about being overheard, run water in the bathroom sink. If you are worried about being seen performing this ritual, lock the bathroom door. Do it; no excuses.

Looking in your mirror, say very clearly and very loudly: "I'm terrific." Repeat it. Your first time will probably leave you laughing self-consciously. You'll get over that by the end of this week. Giggle if you must, but say it at least ten times. Your goal is to look beyond your reflection; you want to look yourself right in the eye and convince yourself from the inside—we'll work on the outside later. Always remember that allure comes from the inner belief you have in yourself. Many women are basically very insecure. Building self-confidence will take time and practice, starting now, with this seemingly silly exercise that actually creates a very solid foundation for your success.

Next, close your eyes and picture the image you'd like to present to the world. You have the potential to become the woman you imagine. Open your eyes and tell yourself that you are on your way.

Gaining Self-Acceptance

Did you know that almost every physical trait can be changed? If you've always wanted blue eyes, you can now have them with special contact lenses. Increased bust measurements are only a silicon implant or two away. Even a weak chin can be remodeled. There are alternatives for nearly every single complaint you might have. But I don't believe this is the only answer.

Some cosmetic improvement is positive: a new makeup palette, a change in hairstyle. But once you begin to remake yourself, you lose touch with who you really are. What happens when you have to take out those blue lenses at night, or when a lover first notices black roots or you break one of the 5″ stiletto heels that compensate for your less-than-statuesque height? Too much trouble.

RULE NUMBER TWO:

Stop being obsessed with your physical appearance.
Start accepting and loving yourself.

But I want to look gorgeous, you are saying to yourself. Yes, do put effort and energy into your appearance, but moderate it. Take good care of your hair and skin: hair that is fresh smelling and caressable is a fabulous asset; skin that is soft to the touch is equally sensuous. Find your best makeup application (see Days 2, 3, and 6) and feel good about it. Making the most of the beauty you were born with is one of the secrets of being alluring, and sticking with the plan means staying alluring. Have fun with makeup, but don't become a slave to your mirror and eye shadow. Don't rush to try every last "look" written up in the fashion magazines—let's face it, beauty editors have to discover new makeup colors and designs every month. But you don't have to wear fuschia and teal eyeliner just because someone photographed it and someone else published it.

Do the most and best you can to highlight your physical attributes and then go on to the more important things in life—you can't forever agonize about not being born Brooke Shields. There will always be someone prettier, no matter how pretty you are. The only answer to this is to be less judgmental and more supportive of the person you are. Yes, prize the physical qualities

---

you have, but more importantly, develop the self that lies within.

> ### RULE NUMBER THREE:
> *If you add attitude and intelligence to enhanced looks, you will be more irresistible than the born beauty and will have a greater feeling of self-worth.*

Nightdreaming: The Second Exercise

Tonight, after you slip under the covers and let your body and mind relax, close your eyes and ask yourself, "What kind of woman do I really want to be?" Do you long to be the seductive type? Maybe you want to be classic, cool, and in control. Do you want a country personality, down-to-earth and completely unpretentious? Do you want to live a life of drama or of quiet evenings? You decide. Try on this new persona in your mind's eye. What kind of changes in lifestyle are needed? Or are you happier, after all, with the life you have now?

Which personality do men prefer? It's not always the sex kitten or the earth mother or any other single type. Men prefer the woman who is comfortable with her *self*, who wears her personality easily and naturally, a woman who is smart and confident, who knows what she wants and has the energy and drive to go after it—the very same qualities you (should) want for yourself.

Projecting the Right Attitude

Thinking positively is step one. Projecting this positive energy through body language is step two. This means acting confident even if you don't yet feel it: head held high, shoulders straight, eyes interested. If you don't believe in the power of having an aura of confidence, take a walk along any busy avenue. Look at the faces of the people around you. Those who are smiling and projecting positive feelings are attractive. Those who have unpleasant expressions and downcast postures make you look the other way. Convinced now?

SUMMARY OF DAY ONE

1. Believe in yourself. Use both the mirror and nightdreaming exercises to build a feeling of self-worth.

2. Project this new confidence with a positive attitude. Think "terrific," and you'll be terrific.

The Allure of the Eyes

T alk to me with your eyes, photographers are forever saying. Sounds trite, but it is true. Your eyes do communicate in many ways. They can suggest a thousand emotions; interest, amusement, understanding, anger, and shock are just a few. Unless you have had professional acting or modeling training, you are probably unaware of the power your eyes hold. Today's exercise will show you how to make the most of this fabulous asset.

A Professional Look

Nearly all initial contact is made visually. When you greet someone, you might shake hands, but your eyes are doing the real work—or should be. Though we think of conversation as verbal, holding another person's attention with your eyes is what gives words their full meaning.

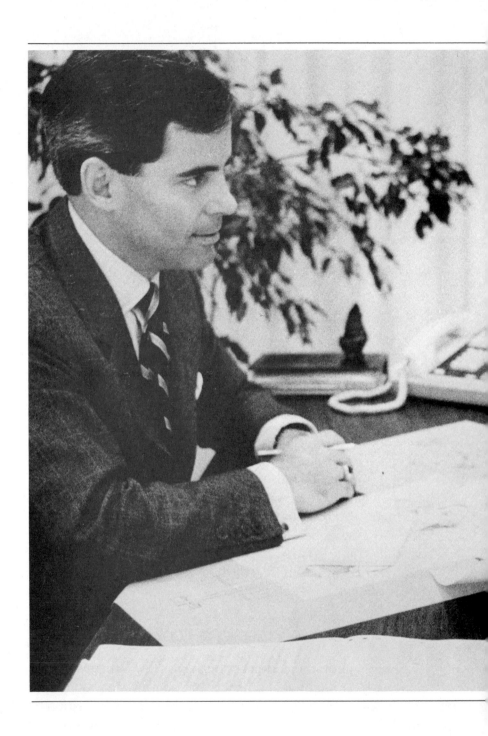

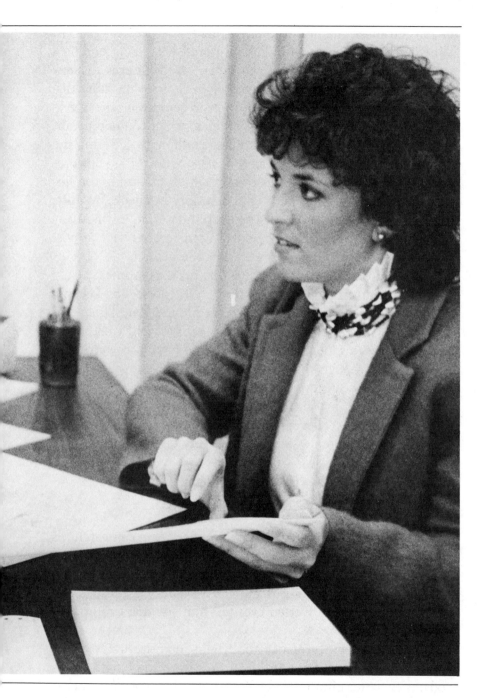

Maintaining eye contact during a business meeting
expresses interest and reinforces a positive first impression.

In business, maintaining eye contact with others is crucial. Whether you are one-on-one in an interview, or are attending a meeting, or taking two clients to lunch, use your eyes to show your interest and earnest feelings. There is nothing more distressing to whomever is speaking than to see the listener's eyes roving. Use your eyes to agree or disagree when you don't want to interrupt with words. Express understanding by lowering the lids as you raise your eyebrows; sympathy by focusing your eyes directly at the speaker's; anger or annoyance by closing the lids to slits or, if you need to keep your emotions in check, by shifting your focus for a few seconds to keep them from instinctively betraying you; astonishment by opening the eyes as wide as possible; disbelief by rolling them towards the ceiling.

If the business situation makes you nervous or uneasy, stop your eyes from darting around—the "shifty" look—by keeping constant focus on the person or people around you. This, coupled with a firm nod to show comprehension, will camouflage your emotions, although you will appear to have a cool attitude. Try to look as though you are in command even if inside you are like a jumping bean: eye control can really help.

Even if you are bored, offer your undivided attention through eye contact; never let your eyes wander to assure yourself a strong degree of professionalism in every circumstance.

The Romance of the Eyes

When you see a man you'd like to meet, you can catch his attention with your eyes. The stare that lasts a bit too long signals your interest. Conversely, when a man doesn't interest you visually, your eyes shift focus immediately; if he tries to catch your attention, your diverted eyes tell him you don't return his interest.

The eyes begin romance, and help intensify it. To tell a man you are attracted to him, your eyes work the length of his body; they flatter him. (Women foolishly feel like objects when a man does this, yet interest is always determined this way. For the sake of curiosity alone, neither sex should blame the other for

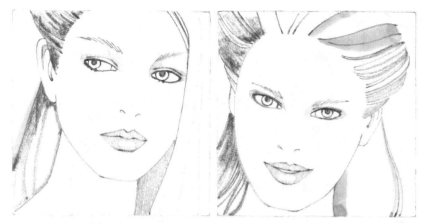

interest   happiness

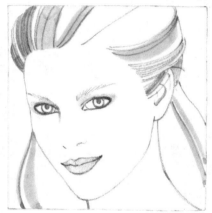

desire

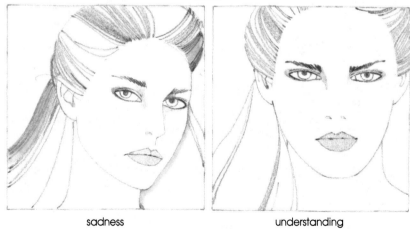

sadness   understanding

The drama of the eyes.

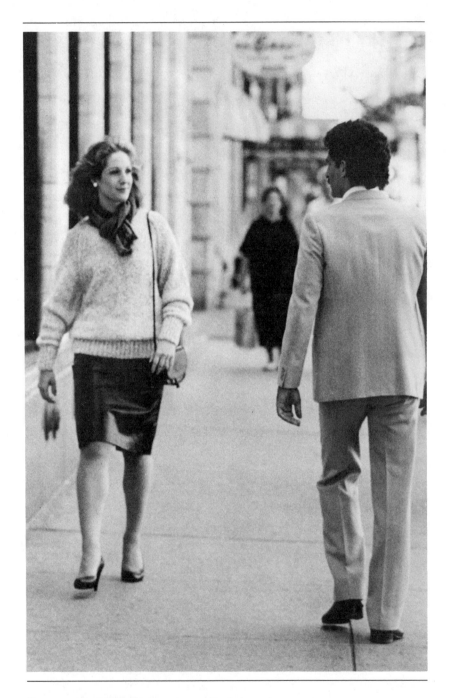

Eye contact initiates a romantic interest
(yes, even on a busy street) . . .

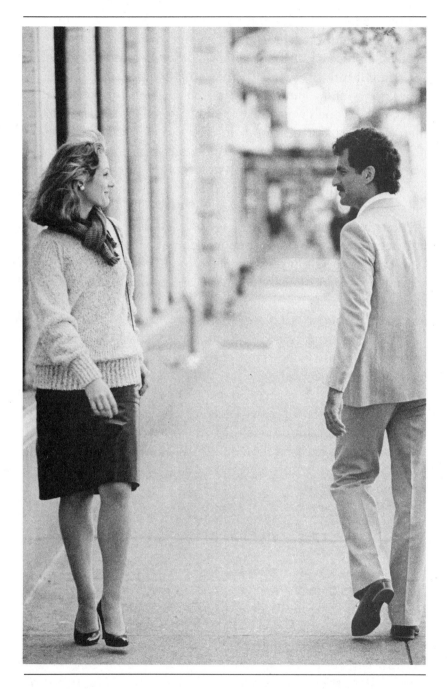

. . . and takes a few seconds to register in this double-take.
If the interest proves mutual, conversation is step two.

taking a good look: this information is seized by the brain and creates an emotional reaction; it is almost involuntary, an unavoidable process. And women do it as often as men do.) Looking straight into his eyes with yours and holding the contact lets him know you are interested and "asks" for an introduction. A quick wink (which women can pull off far more successfully than men) is a great way to return interest a man has shown you.

In romance, maintaining eye contact is also vital. Whether you are on a first date, or celebrating your twentieth anniversary, giving, and requesting, undivided attention strengthens a couple's sense of rapport. Looking down at your hands, even out of shyness, will be misinterpreted as boredom. Use the language of eyes when you want to communicate without words. Slightly downcast "bedroom" eyes that peek upwards through your lashes suggest desire and passion. Batting eyelashes are amusing and can cool a tense atmosphere. A tilting chin and half-closed eyes are an invitation.

Experiment to test the range of your expressions. Stand in front of your mirror and try to convey these emotions using your facial muscles and your eyes: joy, desire, love, sorrow, sympathy and anger. Close your eyes in between to clear away the last image. Finally, evaluate your everyday expression—is there improvement as a result of yesterday's mirror exercise, or does your facial attitude need a bit more uplifting? End this session by projecting a self-confident expression and carry it with you from now on.

The Beauty of the Eyes: Makeup

The basics are few and easily mastered. The most important rule of thumb: make makeup work for you—wear less. Eye shadow (the most misused of all products) and its companion cosmetics are not intended to paint the eyelids, but to make the eyes themselves more alluring. And this requires surprisingly little fuss. Forget everything you've learned about eye makeup till now. Follow these step-by-step guidelines and experiment as though you were applying cosmetics for the very first time.

Eye shadow

Start with a smooth surface by applying foundation or color-less powder over the upper lids; blend well.

Eye shadow is to be used sparingly and only in muted shades: smoky brown, gray, blue, dusty pinks, and mauves. Not bright green, blue, purple.

Neutrals add depth to the lids when applied in the crease of the upper lids. Start the shadow in the hollow above the inner corner of the eye; follow the curve of the crease and end at the outer corner. Use a clean sponge-tip applicator to blend the edges of the shadow into the skin. Best neutral: brown or gray.

Color shadow is applied just above the lashes of the upper lids. Stroke on the barest trace of color. If you like, use it as eyeliner by "wrapping" it around the outer corner of the eye and along the outer half of the lashline of the lower lid. Best colors: muted jeweltones, such as amethyst, sapphire, topaz.

For the browbone (the area from the crease to the eye-brows), forget about using "highlighters," especially those pasty, pearlescent creams. To add a warm glow, use a large soft-bristled brush to lightly apply blusher.

Best overall format for shadows: powder, applied wet or dry, with a brush.

Use a damp cotton swab to remove any flecks of shadow under the eye, then apply a concealer to lighten any dark circles extending outwards from the inner corners.

Eyeliner

Liner can do more than any other product to define the eyes. If you have brown or black eyes, use black liner. If you have light eyes, use a blue-gray or hazel color. A fine-tip brush and cake or a soft, smudgeable pencil works well. Avoid so-called automatic liners in tubes; their consistency is usually too thick to manage.

Apply the liner as close to the eyelash roots as you can. Start at the lower inside corner, using dots that intensify as you near the outer corner. Repeat on the upper lid. Then accentuate the outer corner, or sideways "V" of each eye.

Soften and smudge the liner: a damp cotton swab works on the cake-color; a dry, sponge-tip applicator on the pencil (use the tiniest bit of eye cream on the applicator if needed to avoid pulling this delicate skin).

Mascara

Mascara is magic, but first use an eyelash curler to perk up those lashes. Press gently for five seconds on each side, upper lashes only.

Black is the only true mascara color. There is no single right way to apply it. Start by stroking it on the top side of the lower lashes, then the underside. Next, stroke it on the upper lashes in reverse order: underside, then topside. If the mascara doesn't coat lashes well enough in one application, repeat the steps.

About brands: one claims its tip will distribute color best; another offers adjustable wand positions; a third has a built-in comb to separate clumps. Which is best? Whichever one you work best with. As long as the mascara gets on the lashes, you've applied it correctly. And as for the speck that falls on your cheek, use a damp cotton swab to whisk it away (there is no such thing as no-speck mascara!).

About formats: waterproof mascara has the best staying power, but is harder to remove; use petroleum jelly and do the best you can—you'll lose more lashes trying to get it all off than you ever would sleeping with it on! Water-soluble mascara is better for contact lens wearers because specks that fall into the eyes will dissolve; it rinses off with water, but doesn't stay on as well or as long as waterproof varieties.

1. Learn to pay attention with your eyes when in conversation with others—at business or at play. Do not let your eyes wander.

2. Be aware of the messages your eyes can express. Practice your repertoire of expressions until you master them.

3. Take a fresh approach to applying eye makeup: forget the old rules and try the three-step system outlined above.

The Allure of the Lips

Your lips are an extremely expressive feature, second only to the eyes in intensity—the power of the pout is immeasurable. Lips are beautiful, in every shape and tone. Quite importantly, they reveal your smile. Though you might not be comfortable (yet!) smiling, that is the expression that others want to see. There is nothing alluring about a woman who has, as my father used to say, rocks in her jaws. The look is bitter, and men (and women) steer clear. The fact that you aren't smiling probably has to do with the way you feel about yourself, and that's what needs correcting first. Go and do five "I'm terrific's" in the mirror and then come back . . .

Now that you've started feeling more positive, let me tell you about the lips.

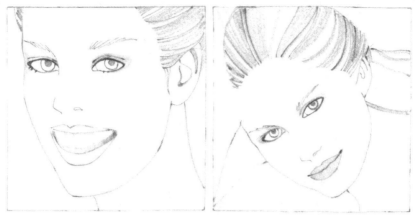

toothy smile   shy, sexy smile

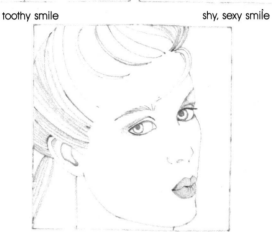

pursed lips

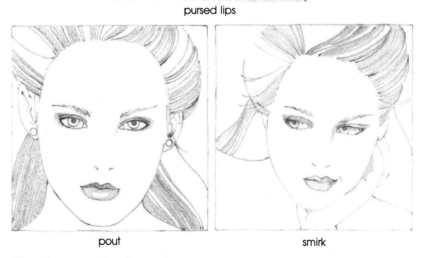

pout   smirk

The drama of the lips.

Provocative Lips

Just as the eyes convey many moods, messages and signals, so do the lips. A wide, toothy smile is friendly, the perfect opener. A closed-lip smile suggests a more serious interest. Purse your lips to chastize, or just the opposite, to blow a kiss. A pouting mouth expresses displeasure in a light way, unless you let it turn into a sulk—and that's completely unattractive.

Test your different expressions and watch your face brighten. Make it the third mirror exercise to add personality and sparkle to your face. The idea isn't to turn you into a coquette, but simply to make you see that your expression is your mirror to the world and the image you want the world to see is an attractive one, to make others stop, look and listen to you. Walking around with a sad or, worse, blank look on your face will cause the world, and everyone in it, to pass you by.

Behind the smile

If the reason you're not smiling has to do with a dental problem, take immediate action. Having perfect teeth is crucial for health reasons, above all others. If your teeth are suffering from a stained build-up of plaque, and if as a consequence, gums are dark, puffy and/or bleeding, see your dentist or a periodontist immediately. If crooked teeth are holding you back, ask your dentist to recommend an orthodontist—it's never too late for braces, and the latest ones practically defy detection. Cosmetic techniques for chipped, spaced and discolored teeth can create the smile you want. And for a healthy mouth, floss every day.

Your Many Voices

Few aspects of a woman are as sensual as her voice. From the coyness of a whisper to the sexy, earthiness of a throaty drawl, the range of voices available to each of us is quite wide. But regardless of the pitch you use, being able to articulate clearly is a priority.

Start with proper breathing to relax you—often anxiety acting on your vocal cords is what makes you sound less than resonant. To establish a regular breathing pattern (essential for exercise as well as general well-being), you must know what correct breathing is. Lie down on the floor, on your back, and place your hands on your abdomen. As you inhale, fill your lungs with air and feel the abdomen expand. As you exhale, draw in your stomach muscles to help push the air out. (Most people do the exact opposite!) Exaggerate the movement of your abdomen until you get used to the direction of the flow of air. Focusing on your breathing will not only help you control your voice, it will help relax you as well.

Next, practice reading aloud. Bear in mind, this is not the time to brush up on your Evelyn Wood reading course. Speak slowly and carefully. Reintroduce yourself to individual syllables and articulate each one with a flourish. Test your range of volume by increasing it a little with each sentence. Stop short of shouting—too much of this can damage vocal cords. Then decrease the tone until you find a well-modulated voice for everyday conversation. For business and casual occasions, your voice should be crisp, quick and clear. A softer, more relaxed and playful voice will be more natural in your private life.

If you are one of the many women who have no trouble speaking until you are faced with a new situation (meeting new people at a party, presenting an opinion at a board meeting, addressing a large crowd), you need to work on building your confidence. Getting over the fear of speaking is best accomplished by knowing you have intelligent things to say. Whether you have to speak in a professional capacity or at an event as private as an intimate dinner, write yourself notes. If you see, in black and white, that you do in fact have something interesting to contribute, you will feel less anxious. Remember one sure thing: others really do want to hear what you have to say and admire those who have the determination to speak up.

For advanced vocal study, try reading from an anthology of one-act plays. Your private performances will help you distinguish your many voices and the literature itself will make you feel smarter and give you great enjoyment.

The Beauty of the Lips: Makeup

Lips are never more provocative than when they are shining with a gloss of color that enhances their natural rosiness. News flash: fuschia, orange, gold and frosted colors, blackberry and sienna do not approach natural rosiness. If, by buying (and worse, using) any of these colors you have committed makeup madness, throw them out at once.

Colors that work include rose; pink (if not too candylike); clear red; coral; wine shades such as burgundy and plum; berry shades that are light, not brown in tone. When selecting a color, be sure to check it in natural light to see if it enhances your natural coloring. Department store lights are rarely strong enough for accurate appraisals. When you shop, carry a good-sized purse mirror with you and go outdoors to check the tested color in sunlight before buying. Remember too that lipstick does not look the same in the tube or on your wrist as it does on your mouth. And one shade will look different on you than on a friend, unless her coloring is identical to yours.

Foundations/Concealers

If your natural lipcolor is uneven, or if your lipline needs added definition, give your lipstick a neutral "base" by lightly applying your foundation or a concealer over your lips and blending the edges into your skin.

Lip pencil

Define and refine the outline of your lips with a lip pencil. Draw the color on the very outside of the line if you want lips to appear fuller; on the very inside to make them thinner. Always accent the center curves of the upper lip. Blend the pencil line into the lips to soften it.

Color

To apply color, some women swear by the lip brush; others stroke it on right from the stick or use a pinkie or index finger. Use whichever method gives you the most dexterity.

Four choices: 1) clear gloss adds shine *only*, great for casual occasions; 2) tinted gloss gives more richness; 3) stick color is for better coverage and formality at the office; 4) stick color plus gloss gives the richest, fullest color, and lots of drama.

Beauty Spoilers

Gum chewing

There is no way to avoid ressembling a cow. NO WAY. And only the cow has the advantage of not looking ugly while she's doing it. Popping gum is also unnervingly offensive.

Smoking

There is nothing sexy about smoke reddening your eyes, rasping your voice and slowly killing you inside. If you need a cigarette as a security blanket, don't light it.

SUMMARY OF DAY THREE

1. Have fun learning the various messages your lips can communicate.

2. Develop your many voices by reading aloud from a variety of sources.

3. Glamorize your lips with color and gloss, always in a shade that enhances, not paints, your natural color.

The Allure of the Hands

Your hands complete the powerful triumvirate responsible for expressive communication. Pretty, well-groomed hands demonstrate the interest a woman takes in her appearance. A warm handshake tells people you are glad to make their acquaintance. Hand gesturing reinforces verbal communication; the physical gesture of touching strengthens a relationship, comforts and reassures.

The Importance of Touch

A popular public service announcement on New York television asks, "Have you hugged your child today?" Children have been found to suffer if deprived of loving touch: their development is slowed; their sense of self-worth, undefined. In truth, everyone longs for the touch of others, from the encouraging "pat on the back" to the tenderness of a lover's hand on the

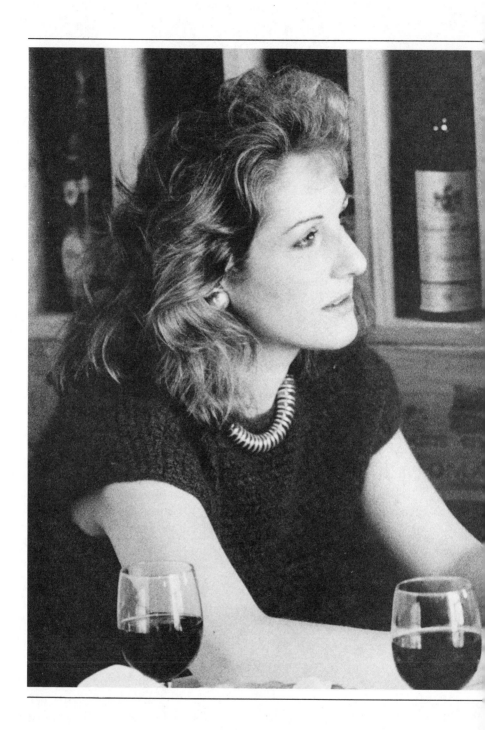

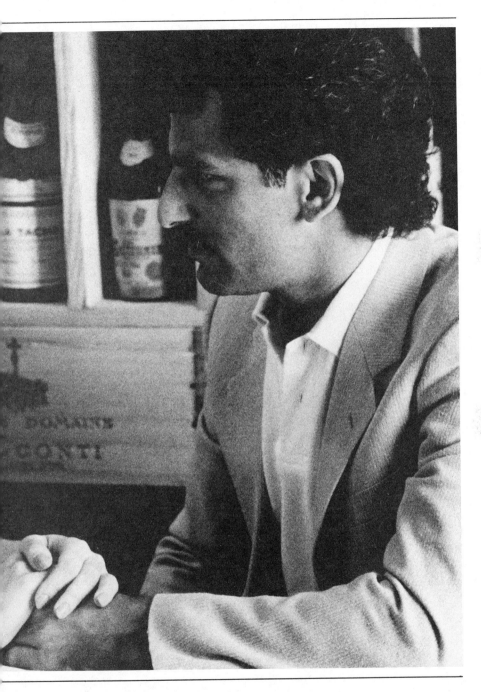

A woman's smile, her eyes and her touch
express growing interest and emotions.

cheek. Perhaps the very power of touch is what makes us fearful of using it to help express our emotions. Yet like all fears, this is one to be conquered.

Little touches make a great difference. A man will hold your hand or put his arm around your waist as a first gesture of growing interest, before a kiss, even before a compliment. To show your interest in him, you might place your hand over his when you are seated, in conversation, at the movies or theater, over the dinner table. Touch his arm to reinforce a compliment or suggestion you offer; his cheek when you are thanking him.

A hug offers more comfort and affection than a thousand words. An arm around his shoulders conveys your message, too. Men adore getting the attention they themselves are expected to give because it is so unexpected. By giving everything you hope of him, you make yourself irresistibly endearing.

One caution: the powers of touch demand temperance. When a strong chemistry exists between you and a certain man, the slightest touch can send sparks flying—one as innocent as a hand that brushes the inside of a wrist. And actions often speak louder than words—be sure yours express what you want them to. If your message is "no," be sure your hands aren't saying "yes."

The Art of Shaking Hands

The one gesture men feel completely comfortable with often gives women the willies. But these are willies easily conquered, out of necessity. If first impressions are made visually, second impressions—just as important—are made when shaking hands.

"But I always shake hands!" you insist. But do you do it well? You must grasp, not grab, the whole hand, so that it locks into yours. (Many people mistakenly take only the fingers in their hands, uncomfortable as well as incorrect.) Practice on yourself—not perfect, but it tops using Rover—until you can locate a willing partner (bankers and insurance salesmen do it best). Hold the hand for at least three seconds, long enough to

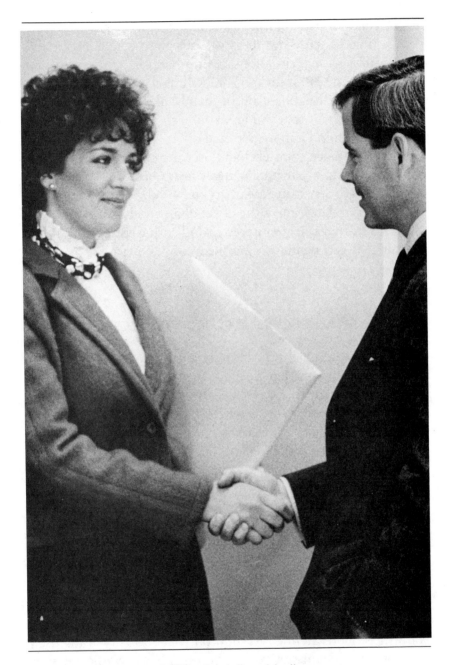

A firm handshake solidifies the interest in those eyes
and that smile. (Fashion note: the bright red
unconstructed jacket formalizes the high-neck ruffled
shirt; the beaded choker adds a hint of glamor.)

tell if it is warm or cold, firm or unsure, and to give the other person time to sense the message your grasp communicates.

In professional situations, a firm handshake conveys interest and earnestness: it says you are willing to do the job and do it well. In social situations, a firm handshake conveys a different kind of interest: it says you are willing to get to know the other person and extend a more personal effort. To express a very special interest, place your left hand over the other person's right as you are shaking. Your hands linger just a bit longer. Your message: "You are a person I want to know well."

Never underestimate the effect of a handshake. At the very least, it says that you are interested and enthusiastic. In its fullest meaning, it can communicate the strongest desires.

Gesturing:
A Misunderstood Communicator

If you were taught at an early age to sit quietly with your hands folded in your lap, you may now unfold them. Whoever first suggested that this was the only polite behavior is probably the same person who first discovered the iceberg.

Because the expressiveness of your hands reinforces the spoken word, gesturing adds credibility to what you are saying. If you are having trouble communicating clearly, gesturing can clarify your meaning. The only caution is to keep your hands away from your face: facial expression counts, too. No matter how shy you are feeling, don't undermine your words by placing your hands in front of your mouth.

The Beauty of the Hands: Manicure

I believe in taking the time to care for your hands because you will be more inclined to show off your efforts by using them in a positive, demonstrative way. Soft hands and manicured nails are the epitome of grace, a lovely quality for every woman to have. This personal grooming takes precious time. However, whether you manicure at home or indulge in a salon visit, the pleasure you will feel at this pampering is more than worth the hour or so it takes.

About the professional manicure. I know one woman who spent a hundred dollars every other week on her nails! She had "tips" put on to increase their length, and did have magnificent hands. But spending this kind of money, even if you can afford it, is certainly not necessary. A new procedure, far healthier for the nails, involves applying a clear protective coating of fibers to strengthen them. Salons often charge $20, but the very same thing can be done at home with a $3 bottle of clear acrylic resin polish, enough for about ten manicures. As you can see, the amount you wish to spend is up to you. Consider your budget. A cost-conscious solution: a professional manicure once a month supplemented by at-home care during the three remaining weeks.

Preparing

Remove old polish thoroughly. Soak hands in a basin of warm, sudsy water. Use a nail brush under each nail to remove dirt. A pumice stone will slough off any dead skin along the sides of your fingers. Finally, rinse hands and dry carefully.

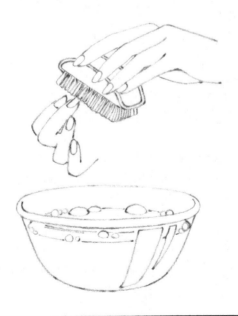

Buffing

To increase circulation and stimulate growth, shine nails with a buffing brush and cream paste, going from right to left only.

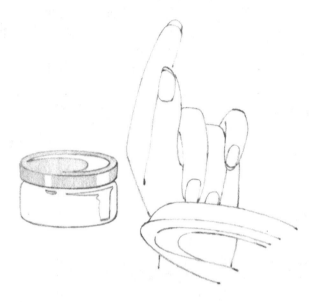

Polishing

1) Using clear polish. Start by using the tip of a white pencil under the nails to brighten them. Next, using clear polish with fibers, paint over the pencil to strengthen the nail and preserve the whitened color. Then apply a first coat to the nail itself, using horizontal strokes. Wait five minutes to dry. Apply a second coat in the usual vertical manner. Wait fifteen minutes, then apply a coat of clear sealer, to protect nails and camouflage the protective threads in the fiber polish.

2) Using colored enamel. Omit the white pencil, but apply the clear polish with fibers both under and on the nail as described above. Wait fifteen minutes to dry completely. Then apply two coats of enamel, waiting fifteen minutes in between. When applying color, do it in three careful strokes: the first starts at the extreme left, the second at the extreme right and

the third, from the center of the nail bed to the tip. When the two coats of color are dry, apply one coat of protective sealer. Do not use your hands for one hour. This waiting time, in between coats and at the end, is the only way to prevent smudges. It does take time, but the look is great. (Sunday night is a good time to give yourself a manicure; be sure to make it the very last thing you do. Also, check and repair chips before bed every night.)

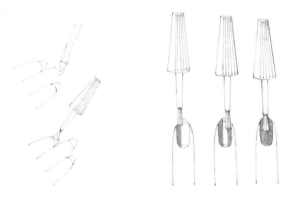

Filing

When the polish is completely dry, file your nails as needed. An emery board won't damage dry polish which in turn protects the nails and makes filing easier.

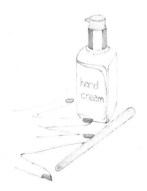

Creaming

Finish your manicure by applying a very rich cream to your hands.

```
┌─────────────SUMMARY OF DAY FOUR─────────────┐
│                                              │
│   1. Recognize the importance of touch and use
│   your hands to reinforce visual and verbal expression.
│                                              │
│   2. Practice your handshake: be firm, yet sincere
│   for successful "second impressions."       │
│                                              │
│   3. Use gestures to help convey your message
│   and to support your ideas.                 │
│                                              │
│   4. To encourage yourself to use your hands as
│   an extension of your personality, keep them lovely
│   and well-groomed. Hands are the perfect    │
│   example of form and function working together.
│                                              │
└──────────────────────────────────────────────┘
```

The Forgotten Art of Comportment

Attitude is present not just in your face, but in your entire being as well. The impression you want to project emanates from your body as well as your facial expression. How you hold and carry yourself is a direct reflection of the way you feel about yourself deep inside. When you see a woman walking with head hung low, slumping shoulders and at a pace that's more of a crawl, your reaction is to look the other way—nothing appealing there. But catch sight of a woman who looks ten feet tall, who wears an expression that says, "I can conquer anything," and you find yourself drawn to that wonderful energy. You might envy it, you might even be angry that she has it and you don't, but clearly you are attracted by it.

Getting Over the Wallflower Syndrome

What she has, and what you want to have, is nothing more

than a feeling of self-confidence well projected. If you wake up feeling great and looking forward to the day ahead (because you have planned something special), you naturally project this energy. But if you wake up feeling sluggish and wanting nothing more than to crawl back into bed, you will naturally project this lethargy. The self-confident woman makes sure she always (well, almost) has a great reason to get up in the morning; she knows how to project "positive" every day, even if forces conspire against her. A woman who can say to herself, "I don't care if it's raining and I have to spend the day canvassing the neighborhood because I know it'll be great," *believes* she can conquer anything. Why does she believe it? Because she has convinced herself. She looks at all she has accomplished and she praises her efforts; she doesn't worry about the mistakes or the failures as many others do.

Too often, a woman tells herself she can't, when she could be telling herself she *can*. We think negatively when we have every reason to think positively. It is time to get over this perverse behavior by simply starting to tell yourself: "Yes, I can do it." Positive reinforcement might sound too simple to be effective. But look how effective negative reinforcement has been in making you insecure and plagued by self-doubt. Simply turn your thinking around.

One important way to project this new thinking is in the way you carry yourself. Your comportment is vital to create the self-confident image of allure. Maybe you do feel just awful one morning, but by projecting appeal on the outside, you are the only one who has to know how you feel on the inside: a must to keep your professional self working, a help to get you to enjoy the personal self. And by putting forward a positive image, you will probably start feeling better sooner.

How Your Body Projects Confidence

If you want to capture attention when you enter a room, you must know how to walk. If you want to be noticed by a special someone in a crowded room, you must know how to stand. If you want to be listened to, at your desk or at a restaurant, you must know how to sit.

We don't often hear the words "comportment" and "poise" used anymore, but having a graceful and commanding stature is what separates the woman who turns heads from the wallflower.

How to stand with authority

1. Relax through proper breathing. Don't allow your body to stiffen. Balance your weight comfortably between both feet; your

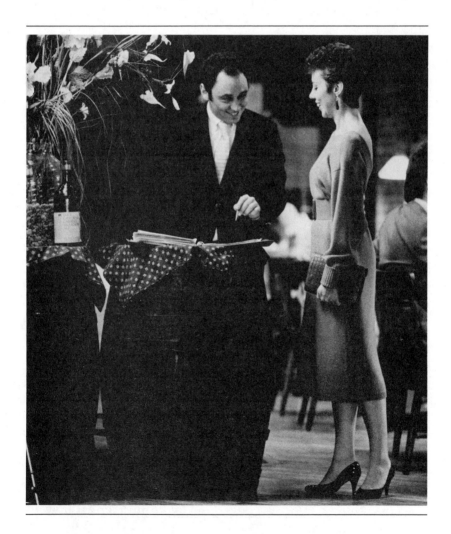

feet should be a few inches apart, one in front of the other. Don't try to stand with your feet together—you'll never be able to hold it, and it certainly doesn't look natural unless you're in uniform.

2. Bring your shoulders back without moving your ribs or back to do it: only the shoulder blades adjust. The line of shoulder-neck-shoulder should be straight, not curved inwardly. Note: if you can't judge how it should feel, lie flat on a carpet and press your shoulders flat into the floor without lifting your bottom.

3. Press your hips forward by tightening your gluteal muscles. You may release these muscles slightly, but don't let your back-side sway.

4. Raise your chin to create a long, graceful neck along with a bit of attitude.

How to walk into a room . . . and turn heads

1-4. See above.
You have to stand before you can walk, right? So start by standing correctly. Walking is the fifth step, not a replacement of any of the others: maintain the "standing" stance as you walk.

5. Lead with your hips, not with your head. It worked for Monroe, it'll work for you. Keep the gluteals tight and put one foot in front of you, a long, graceful stride. Do not be in a rush—how can they notice you if you go by in a blur? Then bring the other foot forward, graceful, measured.

6. Keep your arms at your sides. Do not use them as oars to propel you.

7. While walking into a room with chin raised, let your eyes sweep over the crowd at the doorway or entrance. Take a breath. Take the first stride in. Don't fight your way through a crowd: always stop to let people move out of your way after you've used a firm voice to say, "Excuse me." Getting noticed means allowing time for you to be noticed; that's all it takes to make an entrance.

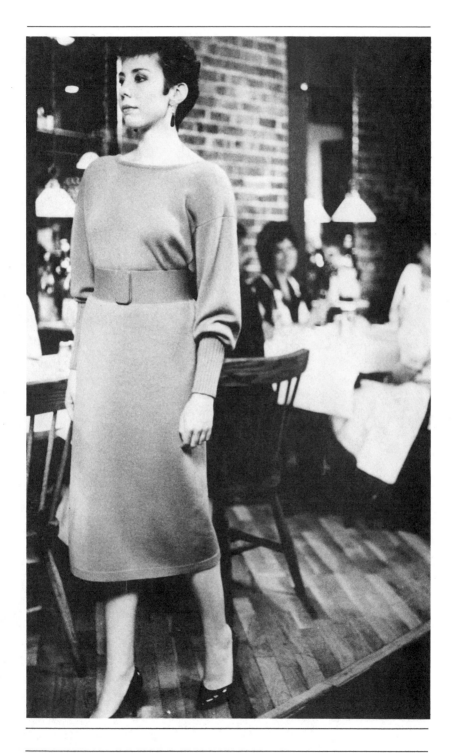

How to sit gracefully

The art of sitting properly is a tricky one; it involves:

1. walking to the front of the chair . . .

2. pivoting so that your back is to it . . .

3. feeling the edge of the seat against the back of your legs . . .

4. lowering your hips to reach it, with a straight back and without collapsing on your hands (tightening tummy muscles helps) . . .

5. and practicing, at home, alone.

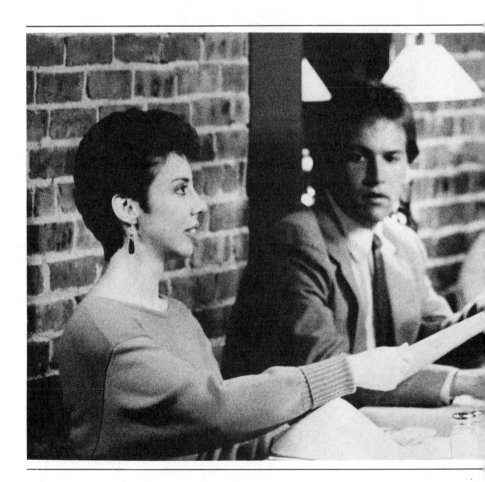

1. Your body reflects your inner attitude as much as your facial expression does: carry yourself as though you are the Hope diamond (or better).

2. Let your actions (the way you stand, walk and sit) project this sense of self-esteem.

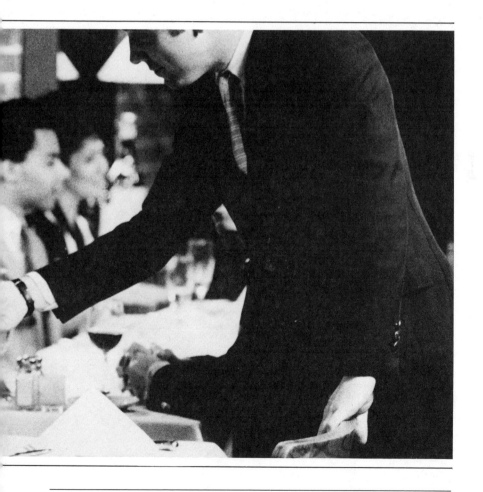

DAY 6

Working with Beauty Flaws

A ssessing your beauty is something you probably can't do with great objectivity, not easily at any rate. You see what you want to see and believe what you want to believe, often becoming your greatest critic and worst enemy. Looking for flaws can become your favorite pastime if you let it.

My own mania centered on my nose. I thought it was too big. And yet I was very often asked for the name of my plastic surgeon—women were convinced I had had it straightened! Who was I to believe? For a long while, I believed my mirror and me. Finally, though, I convinced myself that I was wasting too much time trying to hide my nose and would be far better off if I believed everyone else and left it alone. The unfortunate thing is that no matter how often you are complimented, it will mean little until you start to realize yourself that you truly merit the compliment.

Of course not every flaw exists only in your mind. Some of

your features might very well be better than others. You must try to determine which are the features to be maximized in order to indirectly minimize the others.

Start by applying your best foundation to give yourself a smooth face to enhance. If you don't wear foundation because your skin is excellent, be sure to wash and dry carefully, and blot any oils that create a shine. In either case, applying neutral powder with a large brush will refine the skin further.

Next take a sheet of paper and divide it into two columns. On the left, list assets; on the right, flaws. Give brief descriptions such as "eyebrows: good curved arches" (asset) and "chin: needs more definition" (flaw). Be sure to assess: skin quality, forehead, eyebrows, eyes, cheeks, nose, lips, chin, jawline, ears, neck, and hair.

- Cheeks, eyes and lips should really be considered assets, even if they need makeup: each benefits enormously from makeup.
- Other features can go from flaw to asset with assistance. Tweezers and pencil improve eyebrows; a hint of blush on the chin gives it definition.
- Some flaws can be indirectly minimized. A prominent nose attracts less unfavorable attention when you emphasize cheekbones; a square forehead softens when you wear a hairstyle with bangs. You create the same type of illusion a magician does: to divert the audience's eyes from the trick he wants to hide, he presents something beautiful to look at. Present your audience with exotic eyes and shining lips and they will never see the ears you insist are too large. Remember to *enhance*, not to attempt to camouflage, which is too tricky to pull off.

Maximizing Natural Assets

How to enhance the eyes

Be certain you are following the three-step makeup application outlined in Day 2.

---

1. For close-set eyes, concentrate liner, shadow, and mascara on the outer halves of the upper and lower lids to exaggerate the natural "V" shape. This draws attention to the outside of your face.

2. For eyes that lack depth, wear a rich, deep shadow on the upper lids, and an even deeper concentration of the color in the crease; extend the color halfway to the eyebrows. Use blusher over the upper browbones. Blend the color and the blush so that the edges disappear; use a damp cotton swab.

3. For deep-set eyes, apply a neutral foundation or concealer over the entire upper eyelids to lighten them. Use brown shadow above the crease to the eyebrows. The light color of the foundation brings the lids forward; the dark color pushes the prominent browbones back. If you want to add color to the lids, choose a pale shade. Use lots of mascara to bring the eyes out and into view.

4. For wide-set eyes (every woman's dream), be sure that your liner and shadow start at the inner corners of the eyes to fully define them.

How to enhance the lips

1. Always apply foundation over lips to give you a base; this is vital when using makeup to improve their shape.

2. With a lip pencil, redefine the lips as you would like them. Don't draw a completely new mouth, but do enhance the "M" shape of the upper lip; flesh out thin lips by curving the outside of the natural lipline; widen a small mouth by adding definition to the outer corners. Experiment.

3. Full lips need deep color to minimize their appearance; thin lips need light color to maximize them.

4. Gloss attracts more attention: a must on all but the full mouth which needs only color.

5. Check lipstick two or three times during the day. It gets talked off, chewed off, and sipped off at an alarming rate.

How to enhance the cheeks

1. Be sure your face is clean and prepped with foundation or sheer powder. If you have any bit of oil in your skin, you do not need a moisturizer; this is the most overly touted product around!

2. Have three shades of loose powder: a light color, such as beige; your best rouge, ranging from rose to apricot; a darker shade of the same for contour. The intensity of each shade depends on your skin tone. On pale ivory skin, a medium beige will look dark; on light brown skin, a dark brown will be needed for contour. Why loose powder? You can easily blend your own shades, have more control, and avoid the problem of streaking. Use a medium-to-large brush to apply, not cotton (again, little control), not a sponge, nor a puff which can get dirty and oily. Worried about dry skin? Buy powders that contain oil.

3. The dark, contour shade is applied first. Lightly dust it on under the line of your cheekbones, in a curve, not a sharp diagonal.

4. The rouge shade goes on next, over the fullest part of the cheeks, and is extended into the darker color to obscure it.

5. The light shade is brushed from the sides of the nose across the top of each cheek, past the outer corner of each eye, and then under the cheekbones themselves to soften all edges and brighten the inside of the face. The powders are not intended to re-create your cheekbones, but to define what you have. Always experiment with the placement of color (the rouge, especially): some women look great with a sweep of color that goes from the right cheek across the nose to the left; others look best with color on only the very outside of the cheeks.

"What about my ears?"

Or neck. Or jawline. Or nose. Or square forehead. The lack of perfection in any or all of these is best dealt with by simply accepting the way you are. Example: don't make a concerted effort to hide your ears under your hair. First, the face ends up looking oblong; second, this unsuccessful camouflage announces to the world: "I hate my ears." Sweeping the hair over the tops of the ears, and leaving the bottoms to show, or glamorizing with earrings, works better. When it comes to flaws, this is the one time that leave-it-alone-and-it'll-go-away advice is on the money.

About the neck you hate. Too long? Wear cowlneck sweaters and dresses. Never tie a scarf around it—that's from the waving-a-flag school. Too short? Wear jewels, and V-necks.

About the jawline. A sculptured jawline is great—not as angular as you might fear. Long hair will detract from it, if you insist you hate it. A round jaw or weak chin straightens up with a short, angular haircut; emphasizing cheekbones "corrects" roundness; a touch of blush defines that chin.

About the forehead. Squared corners can be softened with bangs or a stroke of warm brown or rouge powder. Bangs work on even a low forehead if they are cut from the crown.

About that nose. As a constant experimenter with shading, I say leave it alone. (I must add that I reached this conclusion only after my brother-in-law Phillip asked one day, "What are those brown marks on the sides of your nose?") If you are worried about the appearance of your nose in a photograph, then you might use a brush to lightly stroke brown shadow on the sides, and a soft line of neutral color straight down the front. But wash it off before you leave the photographer's studio because in natural light, it will look like the side view of an Oreo cookie.

About skin quality. The truth is, aside from keeping skin clean, there's little you can do. Skin will blemish until the body tells it to stop. It will look sallow if your DNA programmed it to look sallow. You will break a few capillaries and develop dryness or lines (which a light cream can help minimize). You can improve the *health* of your skin through nutrition, lots of exercise, eight glasses of water, and eight hours of sleep every day. But for a flawless look, you will need a good foundation: oil free if you have oily skin (Janet Sartin's "colored astringent" is the best), or with a minimum of oil if you have average-to-dry skin (the lighter the preparation the better). Apply two light coats rather than one thick one if you need extra coverage. Then brush on the sheerest translucent powder for a terrific texture.

Only a handful of women have naturally flawless skin—too few, in fact, for you to waste time envying.

About your hair. There are no two ways about it: your hairstyle can make or break your look. The Catch-22 about hair: there's little you can do. Notice I said "you." In the hands of a professional, anything is possible.

Calling In The Professionals

Want the one beauty secret that will forever free you from roaming the counters at your favorite cosmetics store? If you feel that your own efforts are not accomplishing enough, get the advice of professionals. In the hands of a skilled makeup artist and a talented hairstylist (a good number do both), you can achieve fabulous results.

An independent makeup artist, hired by you, has your best interests in mind; he/she is more concerned with enhancing your looks than with selling you a line of cosmetics, or with making a statement on your face.

A hairstylist, though often connected with a salon, also has you as the number one priority: he/she wants you to be a regular client and will put your needs above an urge to "create."

Finding a beauty professional is not as hard as it sounds. The first place to look is the cover credit page of your local magazine or newspaper magazine section, provided you like the way the cover models look. Next check out the appropriate credits at the end of locally produced television shows. Once you have two or three names, do a little phone work. Call to see if they take on private clients, how much time they will devote to the appointment, and how willing they are to discuss your specific requests. At your session, resist forcing the use of your present cosmetics. If you've chosen the wrong colors or formats, force yourself to throw them out and start from scratch.

If the makeup artist doesn't do hair, ask for his/her recommendation of a salon stylist or an independent. For more on hair, see Day 12.

Why do I strongly recommend putting your beauty into a professional's hands? Because no makeup chart or book of hairstyles (not even one written by one of these experts) can possibly take into account those millions of feature characteristics that exist and that make each woman an individual. Because a trained, skilled pro can see you in a positive, yet critical way that neither you nor your best friend can. Because the results will be immediate and long-lasting and will save countless hours of trial-and-error experimenting (fun at the beginning, exasperating after a few sessions) and hundreds of dollars—even if every five years you make another appointment to appraise the changes in your face. Best of all, it will free you from beauty bondage to concentrate on the inner you.

When Should Plastic Surgery Be Considered?

On turning thirty-five, my friend Betsy finally came to a decision she had been wrestling with for ten years. She decided to have the unsightly bump in her nose removed. During her consultation with a surgeon, he suggested another procedure which he believed would have tremendous results, a chin implant to improve her undefined jawline. Betsy made this her very special birthday present.

Before her surgery, Betsy was not the attractive woman she is now (note that she is still not model-beautiful), but she did have a good self-image. She was vital, vibrant and confident. The surgery meant putting the finishing touches on a great person, not creating one—surgery can't do that. What it can do is simply improve your appearance.

Consider plastic surgery if you have a strong physical need for surgery; if you feel a professional medical opinion is needed; or if you want to present an outer image that better reflects your inner self. The results can be dramatic. But promise yourself this:

if the doctor you consult tells you he sees no real need for any procedure, believe him.

SUMMARY OF DAY SIX

1. Learn to temper your naturally overcritical nature and to appreciate your natural assets.

2. Ignore weak areas and maximize eyes, lips and cheeks until they are distinctively beautiful. Relearn makeup techniques TODAY.

3. If you aren't happy with your own results, turn to the experts for an individual make-over: the best beauty investment you can make.

Three Beauty Makeovers

Every woman has the potential for great beauty. Makeup highlights individual features; hairstyling frames them. The following makeovers show you step-by-step transformations. The photographs, large and clear, tell the story: there's no hidden magic, just skill of application (the techniques are described in the preceding chapters) and the all-important tailoring of makeup placement to each face. You add the desire to experiment as you use this portfolio to inspire you to find your best face.

I. Elaine.

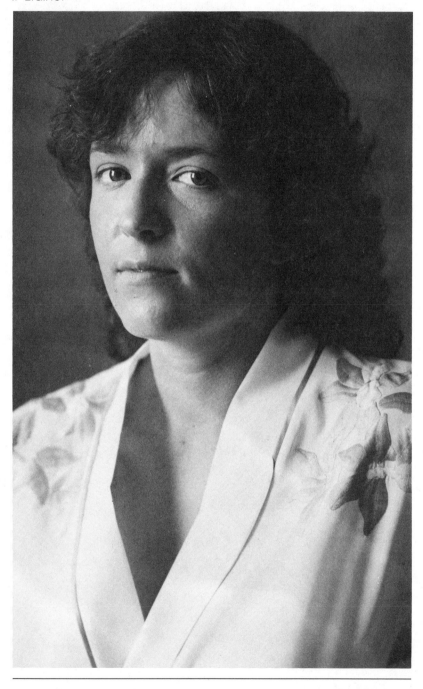

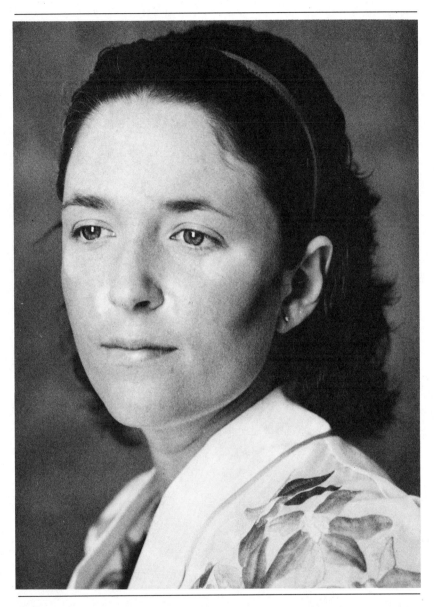

A water-based foundation is best for Elaine because her face is oily. Next, concealer is applied: around the nostrils, the outer corners of the mouth and under the outer corners of the eyes to the top of the cheekbones to create a better contour. Right under this diagonal line of concealer goes a streak of blush and, below that, a deeper blush that acts as contour. Apply all three "cheek colors" before any blending.

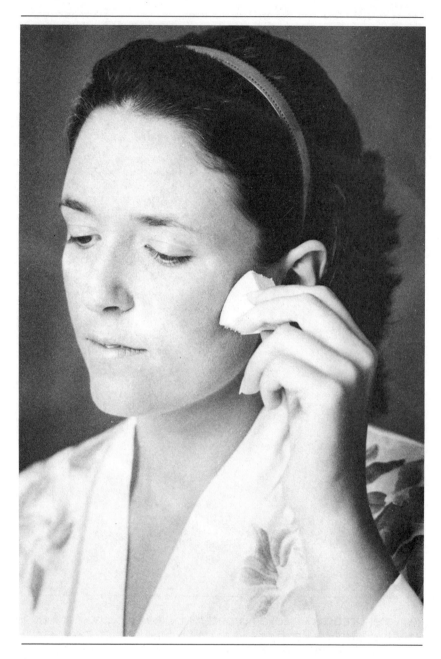

Blending is done from the hairline toward the center of the cheeks. Here, Elaine uses a triangle of a makeup sponge. Next, the sponge is used to bring the cheek color around the temples to soften the forehead.

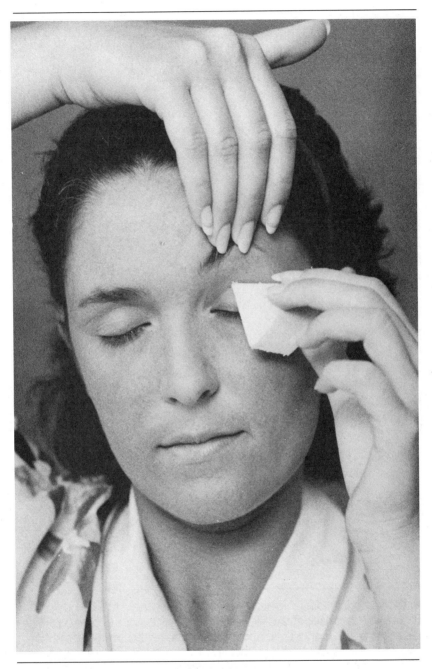

Translucent, no-color powder is applied, using
another triangle of sponge. Applied over the face,
especially the eyelids, it "sets" foundation and blush.

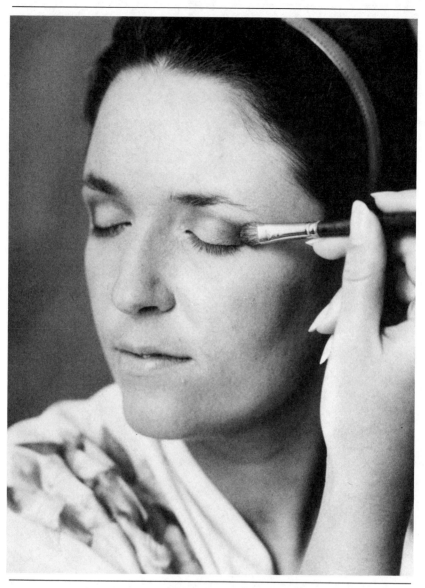

After applying pink highlight shadow over the browbone, Elaine emphasizes the crease in the eyelids with a deep plum-prune shade. The application starts *above* the inner corner at the browbone and follows the line of the bone to the outer corner where the shadow is more concentrated. (Close your eyes and feel the browbone before you apply color to get a better sense of placement on *your* lids.) Next, the crease color is blended into the highlight to obscure demarcation lines.

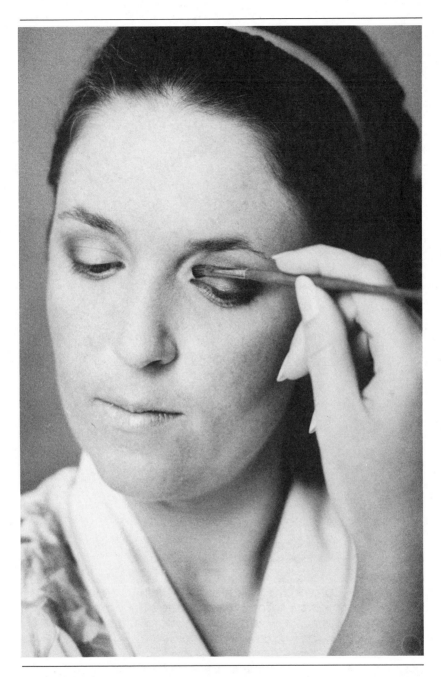

To slim the nose and make the eyes more prominent,
white shadow is applied at the inner corner of
the eyes, blended into the crease color.

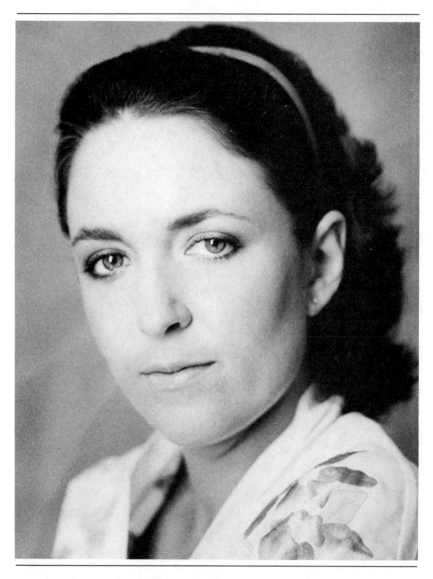

To complete Elaine's eye makeup, a very thin brush is used
to dot the slightest bit of the crease shade on the other
side of the white shadow, at the very base of the bridge of
the nose. A dark gray-plum pencil lines the eyes (upper and
lower lids) and is blended with a narrow brush. Mascara
and a few strokes of brown eyebrow pencil to define Elaine's
brows complete her day look. For drama at night, green-
gold shadow is used on the lids, with more pink highlight
shadow on the upper part of the browbone.

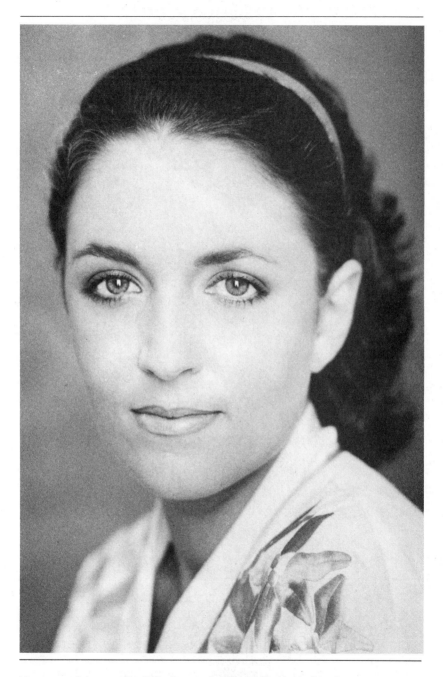

Lip pencil is applied to the outside of Elaine's lips to make them fuller. After lip color is applied, concealer dabbed on with a cotton swab refines the lipline, as needed.

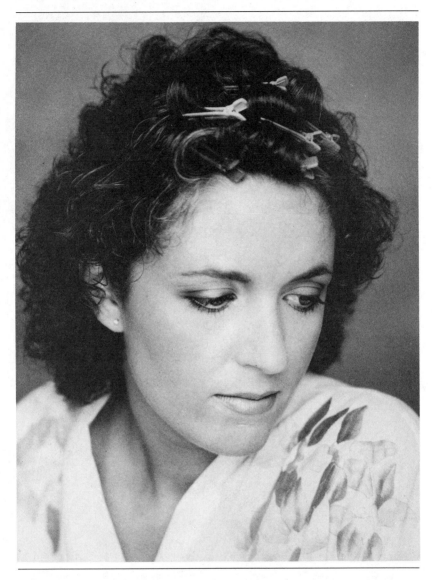

Elaine's hair was cut in the back because that length was pulling down her face. Light bangs around her face and the new added fullness at her neck also accentuate her eyes. Because of her hair's natural waviness, only the front needs setting, for height. After applying setting lotion, Elaine sections her hair, pulling each up from the scalp and then rolling it back, pinning through the curl, not fastening it flat against the head. Note that Elaine used imperfect sectioning to avoid having the hair part unnaturally when dry.

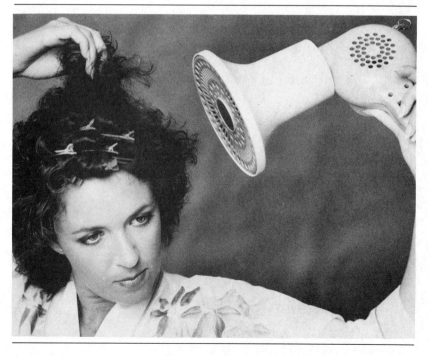

After spraying setting lotion over the rest of her
head, Elaine dries her hair using a diffusion attachment
to gently dry without blowing out natural body.

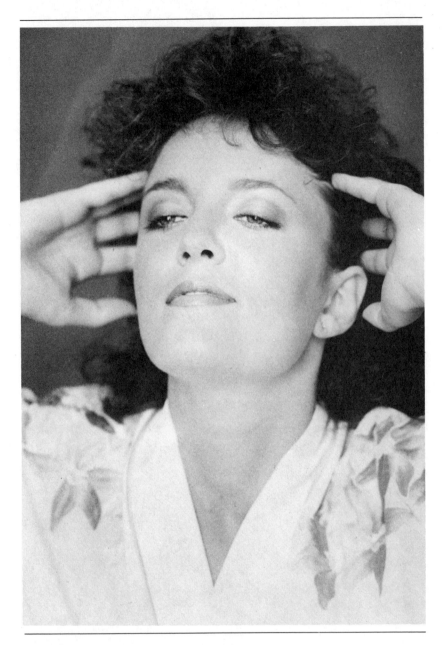

Elaine's "comb-out" is done with fingers,
not a brush. After applying hair spray, she uses
fingers to direct the hold. Light teasing with a
comb adds volume. Directing those little wisps
across her forehead softens the look.

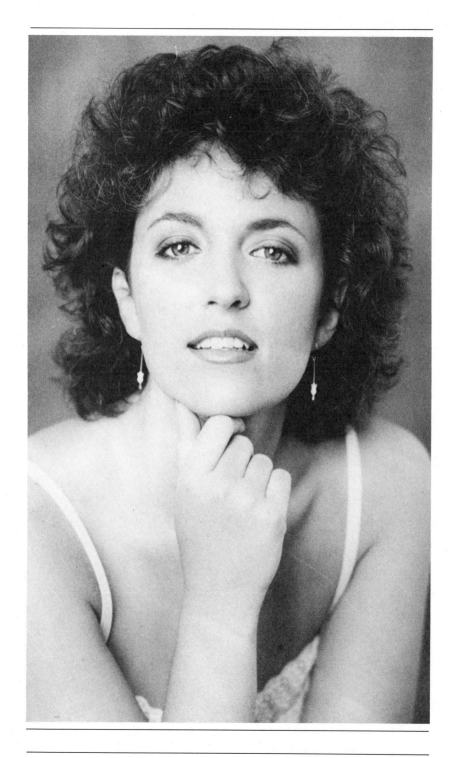

II. Annemarie.

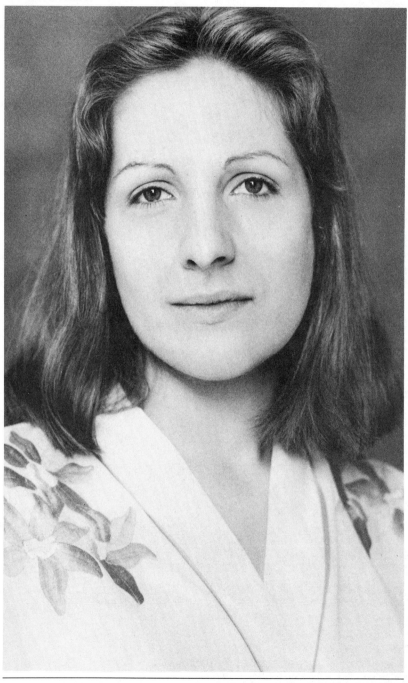

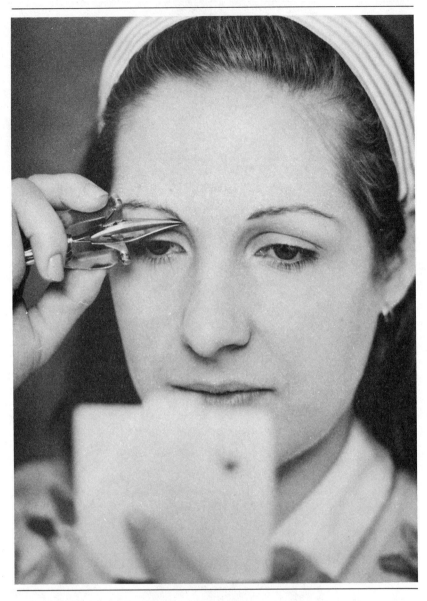

Before any makeup is applied, eyebrows need to
be groomed. Annemarie's brows are too thin before
the arch yet also start too close to the eyes.
Tweezing (done here with a professional makeup
artist's tool by Soligen for less ouch!) removes
the hooks on either side of the nose. After the
skin has a chance to rest, foundation is applied.

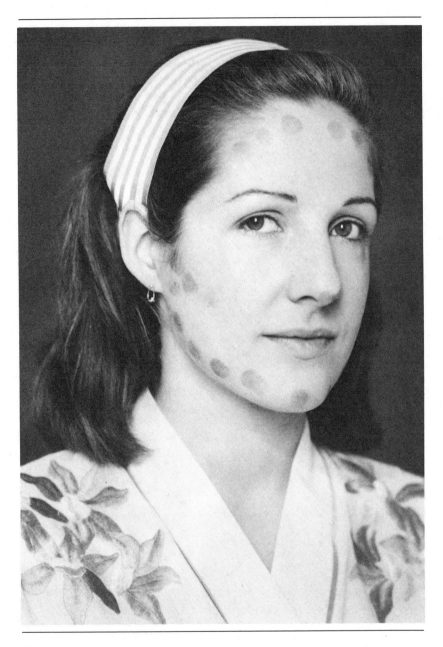

Dots of cream blush act as contour to
trim Annemarie's long face. Color is used to
soften the jawline and the forehead, to
highlight cheekbone definition and to bring up
the slight hook of the nose.

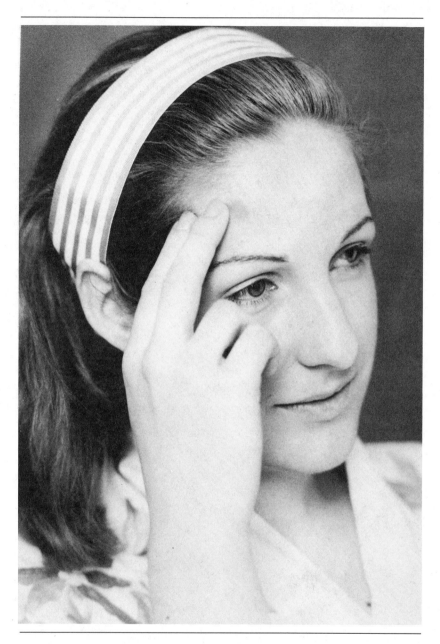

Blending is done by making little circles
with one or two fingertips. After all the dots are
blended, more color is added to the cheeks
proper. Light concealer on the very top of the
cheekbones is used to bring them into focus.

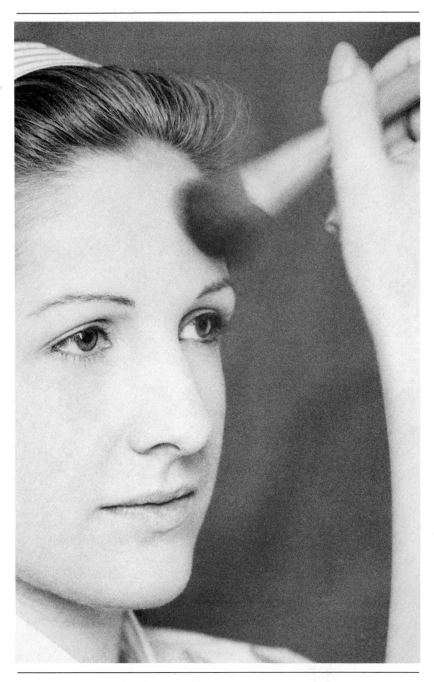

Annemarie uses a large brush to apply cornsilk powder over her face, a boon to skin prone to perspiration.

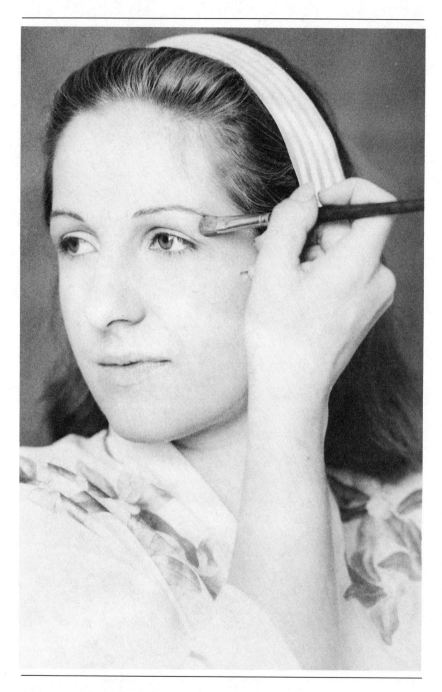

A deep amethyst shadow "pushes" the browbone
back to de-emphasize it.

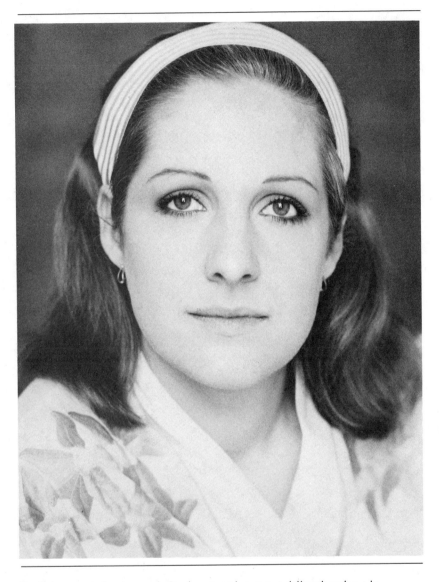

To bring out Annemarie's deep-set eyes, white shadow is applied over the lids. A wine shadow emphasizes the creases and the outer corners. Violet pencil acts as eyeliner on the upper lids. On the lower lids, gray pencil is drawn on the inside as well as the outside to define and open the eyes. Again, additional color, from the liner pencil, is used to accent the outer corners. Mascara is meticulously applied to each lash, upper and lower lids. A light eyebrow pencil adds fullness while Annemarie waits for brows to fill in naturally.

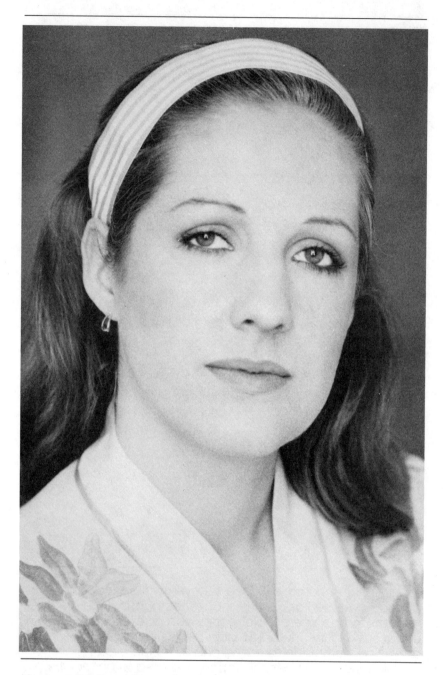

Lip pencil follows the natural curve of
Annemarie's lips, then a pink-lilac creme fills
in with color to complement her blond hair.

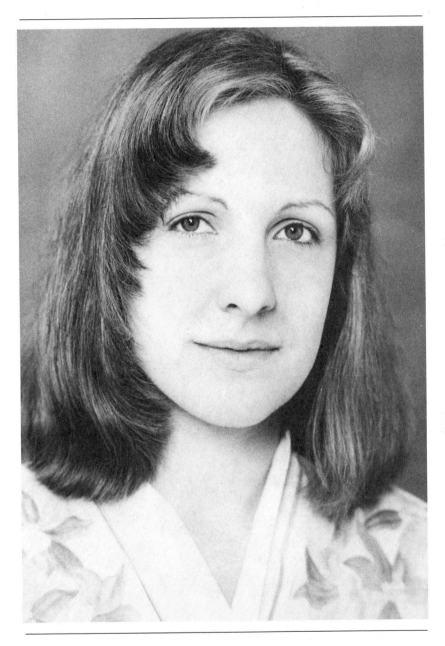

Before her makeup was applied, Annemarie's
hair was shaped. Here, you can see the difference:
light layering in the front softens the long
line of the face and gradually blends into
the long, blunt cut of the back.

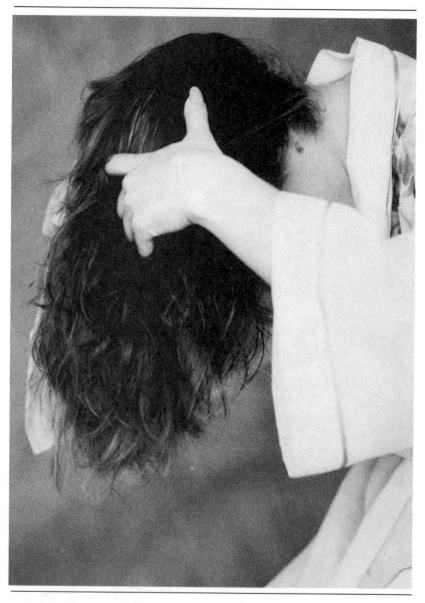

Volume can be added to Annemarie's hairstyle without rollers. With her head hanging over, she directs her hair away from the scalp. When the hair is dry, she sprays on setting lotion and uses a curling iron to add waves to those layered ends in the front. Her finished tousled look is achieved with light teasing and using fingers to direct those wisps across her forehead.

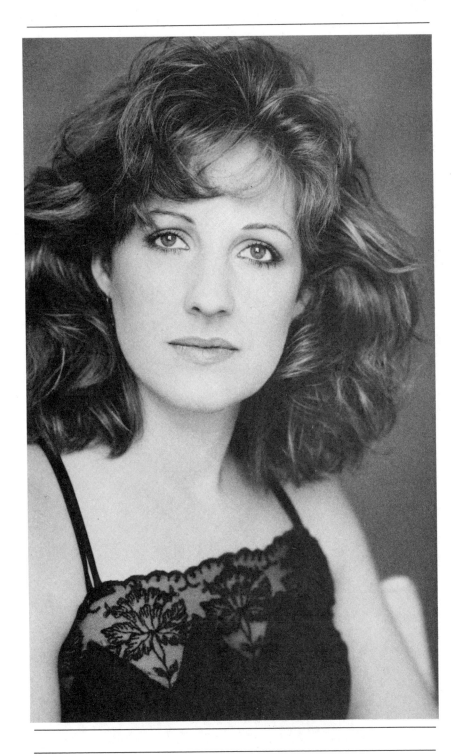

III. Michele.

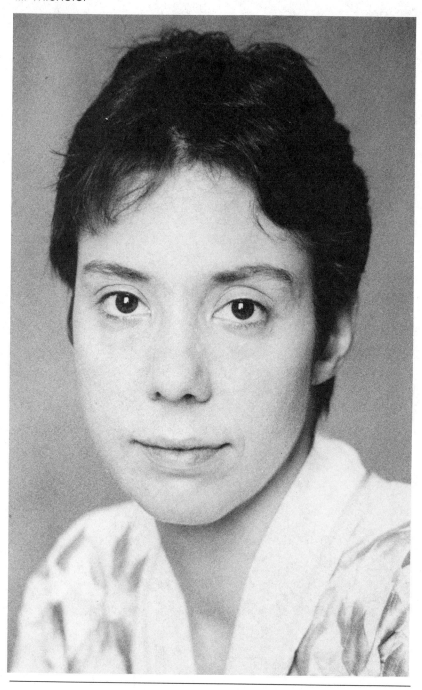

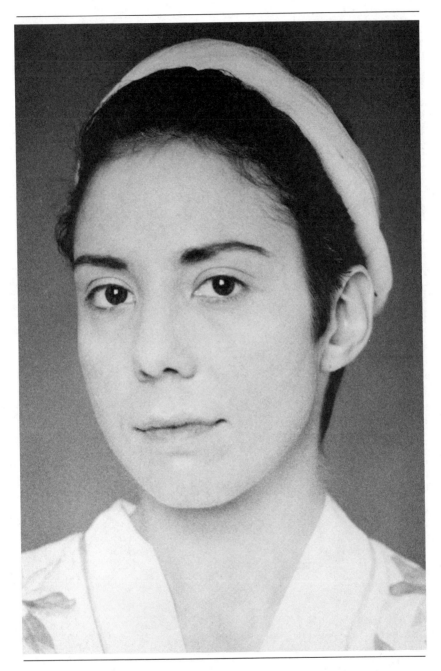

Michele's eyebrows needed a different kind of attention:
thinning after the arch. Tweezers refine the good line
of her brows; a few strokes of pencil fill in light areas.

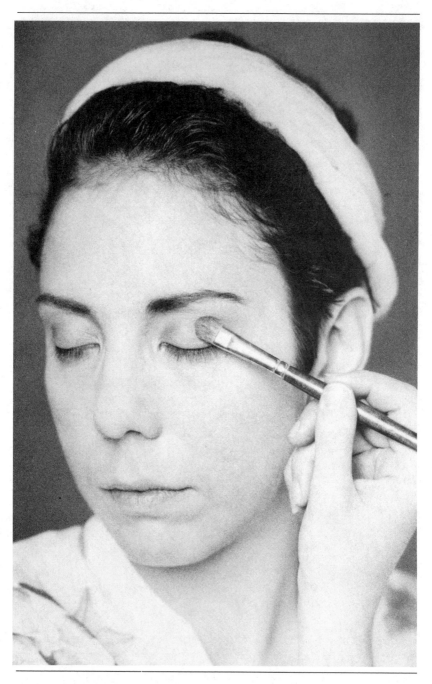

After applying a navy shadow in the crease, Michele
strokes plum color on the eyelid, blending carefully.

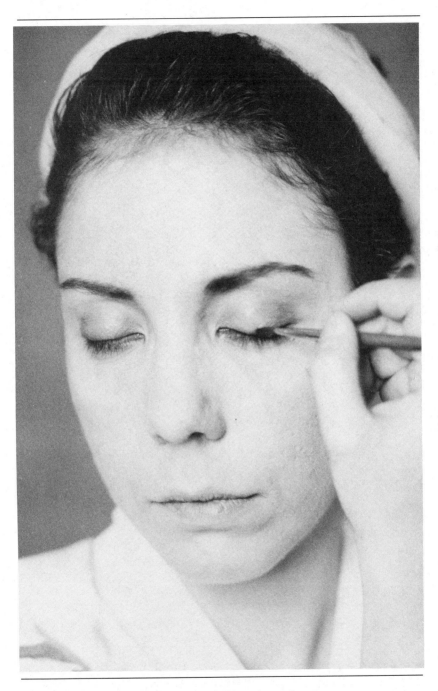

Teal eyeliner is blended along the lashline with
another brush (a cotton swab is an alternative).

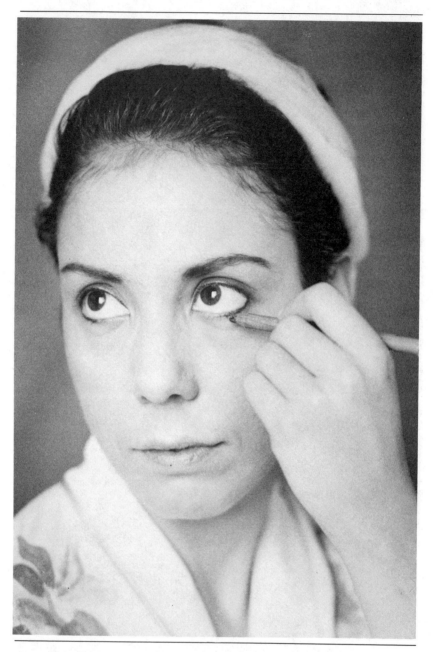

The same teal pencil is used to define the lower
lashline (always work from the outer corner in). The
greatest emphasis is at the outer halves of the
lashlines. Again, the pencil line is blended with a brush.

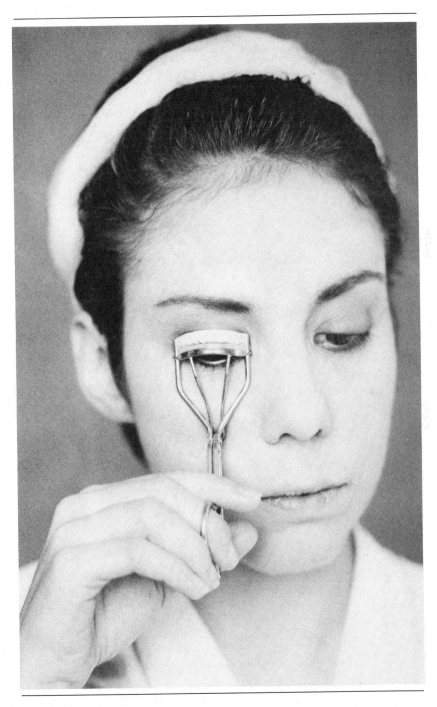

The eyelash curler is indispensable!

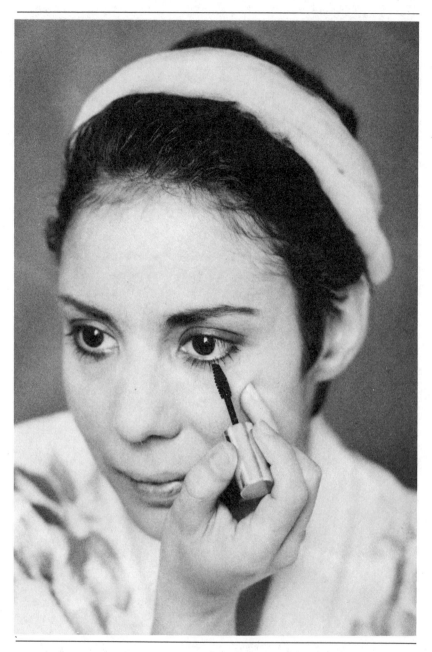

Mascara is applied to *lower* lashes first: looking down can cause top lashes to press against lids—wet upper lashes would smear a great eye shadow application. By holding the wand perpendicular to the lashline, Michele covers each lash.

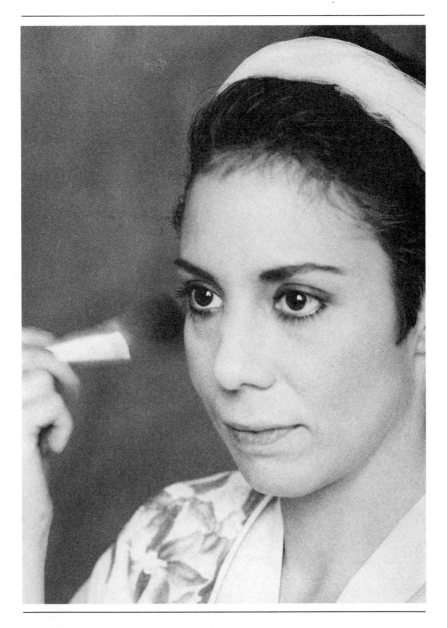

Powder blush works best on Michele's oily skin. She applies
it with a flurry of quick strokes starting at the hairline,
coming in toward the center of the cheeks, then around the
temples and across the forehead. This wide brush works
terrifically. Deeper, contour color is stroked on the same
way, following the curve of the base of each cheekbone.

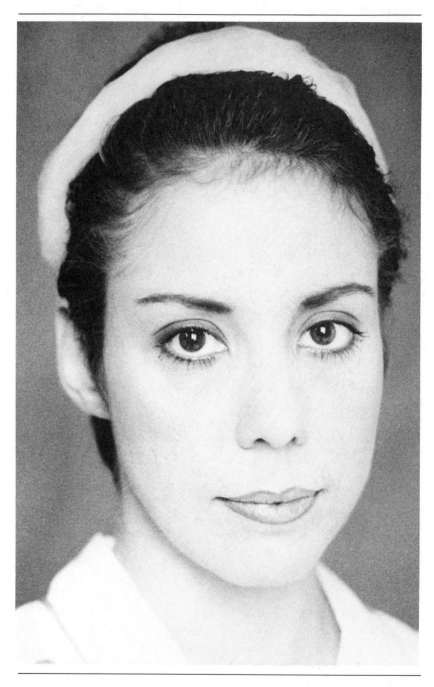

Lip pencil defines Michele's sweetheart-shaped mouth—
notice how the pencil reaches all corners.

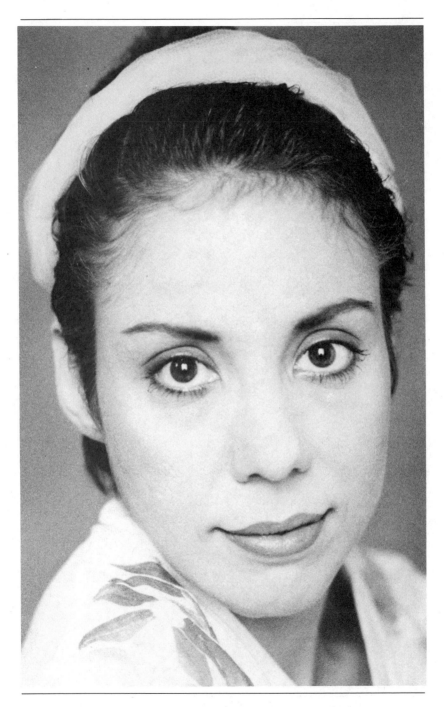

Lipstick gives rich color . . .

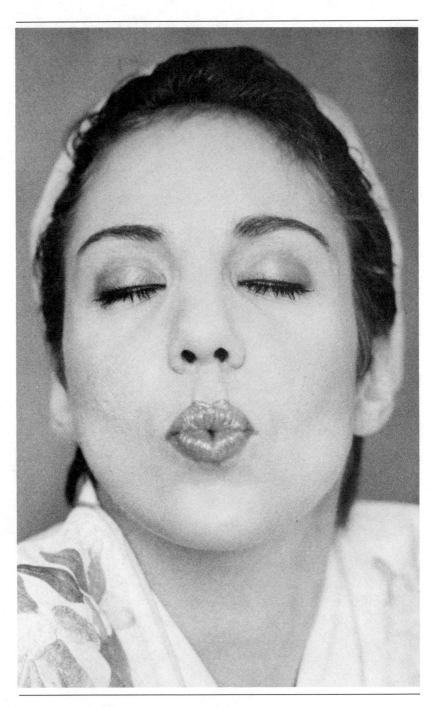

. . . and lip gloss makes lips fabulously kissable!

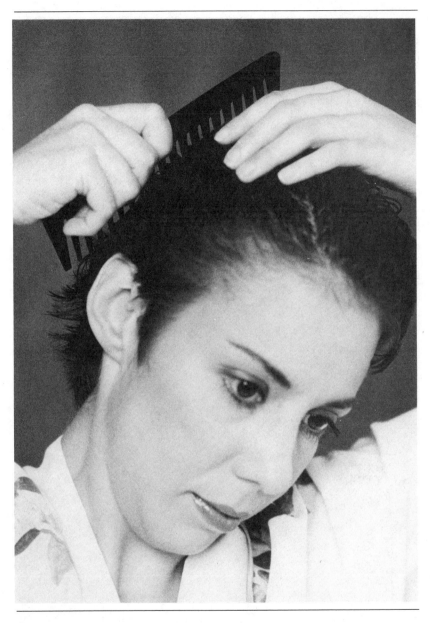

Michele's fine hair lends itself to a short style,
but need never look mannish. The sides and back are
combed into place, sprayed with setting lotion
and allowed to dry naturally. Using a curling iron or making
small pincurls gives height at the crown and a few bangs
pulled out and over the forehead add softness.

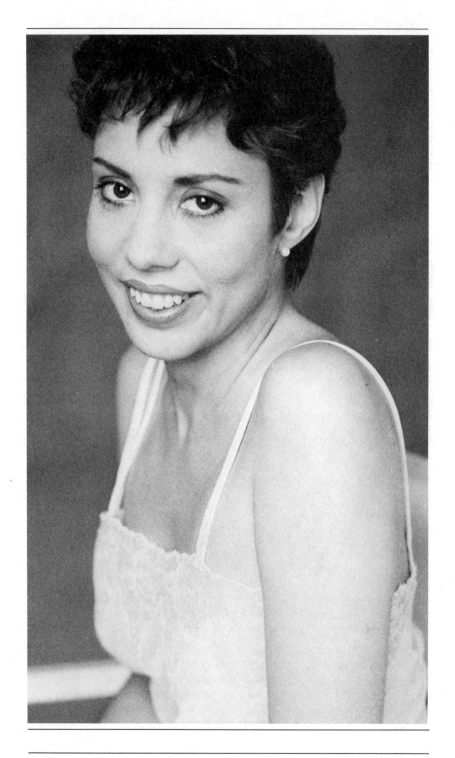

DAY 7

Putting Beauty to Work for You

Organization

To accomplish a job and reach a goal, you must have organization. The following schedule is designed to fit ongoing practice of this week's concepts into your everyday life.

DAILY ALLURE RITUALS

exercise	*time allotted*
Mirror exercise: "I'm terrific"	3 minutes to psych yourself at the start of the day, EVERY DAY
Expressiveness training: eyes/lips/hands standing/walking/sitting	1 minute on each

---

Nail check and chip repair, if needed	10 seconds to 5 minutes (drying time)
Makeup application: note: a young face needs more to add interest; a mature face has its own magnificent depth, and needs less	15 minutes maximum
Nightdreaming: reinforcing self-esteem	5 minutes or until you fall asleep

WEEKLY ALLURE RITUALS

the effective manicure	up to one hour
voice training: reading aloud	half-hour (or five minutes every evening)

Clean Sweep: Evaluating Your Cosmetics

New makeup techniques lose their value if the cosmetics you apply aren't up to snuff. If the format is wrong—example: a gel rouge instead of sheer powder, you won't look as great as you could. If the color is wrong—a murky oxblood lipstick instead of a clear red, you won't look as great as you could. Many women will keep using the wrong cosmetics out of force of habit. Time to evaluate your collection.

Clear off a desk or table, preferably near a window. Have a large mirror handy. Next gather every last cosmetic: retrieve items from purses and shoulder bags, the medicine chest, your desk drawers, pockets of coats—everywhere you might have stashed a lipstick or a compact. Separate the items by category

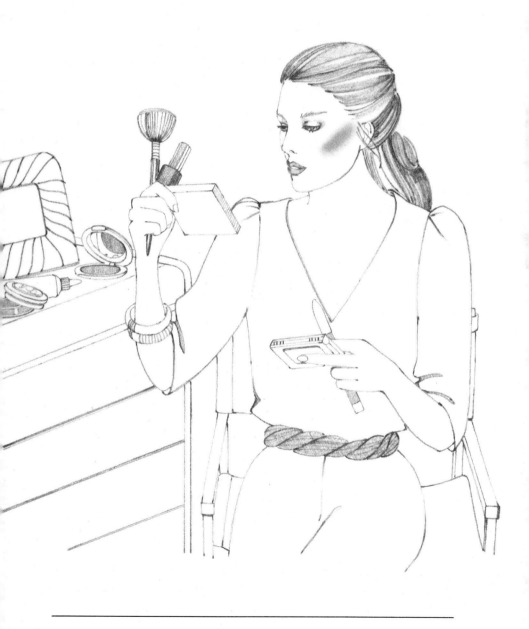

(shadows; lipsticks; etc.). Lastly, apply foundation or sheer powder, just as you did on Day 6, to give you a clean "canvas" to work with.

Not everything must be tried on. Automatically THROW OUT any item more than a year old or that hasn't been worn in more than six months. Pare down to the freshest items.

Check condition

- Check the condition of each mascara on the wand. If it is moist and glossy, put it in the "keep" corner. If not, it goes in the trash.
- Check the condition of sponge-tip applicators. Are they too dirty to apply true color? If so, out they go. Most brushes can be washed; first stroke each back and forth on tissue to remove excess powder, then swish them through a basin of mild soap and water; let dry in a well-ventilated room to avoid mildew.
- Check the rubber strip in your eyelash curler; if the rubber is nicked, replace it.
- Check the cleanliness of cake-powder shadows and blushes. If oils have "dirtied" them, try using a small knife to cut off the top layer and expose fresher powder. When buying new cosmetics, choose loose powder whenever possible (many stage makeup shops will sell loose eye shadows as well as rouges).
- Sharpen all makeup pencils for the most accurate application.

Color test

Once you've checked the condition quality of the cosmetics, you must check the color quality to determine whether or not each item enhances your natural coloring. How fresh the makeup product is or how good it looked in the store doesn't matter if you don't look great wearing it now.

Start with eye shadows. Have plenty of tissues, eye cream (for easy removal of shadow) and cotton swabs at hand. Using the techniques described on Day 2 and Day 6, try on each shade, one at a time, carefully removing each color before applying the next. Each time, ask yourself: does the color enhance my eyes? If it does, put the shadow in the "keep" corner. If it doesn't, throw it out; do not think twice.

Next play with rouges and blushers using techniques described on Day 6. If you have loose powders, or cakes that easily "powder," use a wide brush and a bowl or container to blend your own variations until you find one you like. When evaluating a cheek color, consider the indirect effect it has on your skin. Take an overall view of your face from at least one foot away. Does the color make your skin look yellow? ruddy? dull? If the answer to any of these is yes, the color is not for you. If you can't alter it using another color or a neutral (to lighten it), throw it away.

Lastly, try on your lipstick shades using techniques described on Day 3 and Day 6. Remember to enhance your natural color, not mask it. If the color is too dark, it makes the mouth look like a wound. If it is too light or frosted, it makes the face look pasty. Think, and wear, *bright*.

Take an inventory of the items in the "keep" corner and compare it to the list of cosmetic essentials. Fill in your makeup wardrobe as needed.

MAKEUP ESSENTIALS

cosmetics	companion products
foundation	application sponge or cotton
concealer	moisturizer for thinning it (for easier application)
loose powders: • sheer, neutral shade to prevent shine • light, to highlight (a flesh tone, not white)	two or three brushes of varying width

- rouge for blushing
- darker rouge for
  subtle contour

eye shadow:
- color for interest
- neutral for depth

brushes or sponge-tip
  applicators
cotton swabs

eyeliner

brush if using cake

mascara

eyelash curler

eyebrow pencil, if needed

eyebrow brush; tweezers

lip pencil

lipstick

lip gloss

optional: application
  brush(es)

plus: all items needed for
      a complete manicure; soap/
      cleanser for skin care;
      eye cream for under eyes

WEEK TWO

Style

S tyle is image. First, knowing what image you'd like others to see. Second, projecting it. Unlike beauty, it's not something you are born with. It is a sense of taste acquired while you were growing up or developed as an adult. Style is not money. In fact, having a sense of your own style enables you to stretch a small budget and work with what is available to make you look your best. Anyone can wear a designer dress—style makes it look more your own, and can turn an inexpensive dress into your own "designer" original.

This week is designed to show you how to express yourself through your clothes and your surroundings, to get you in touch with yourself and the image you want to project.

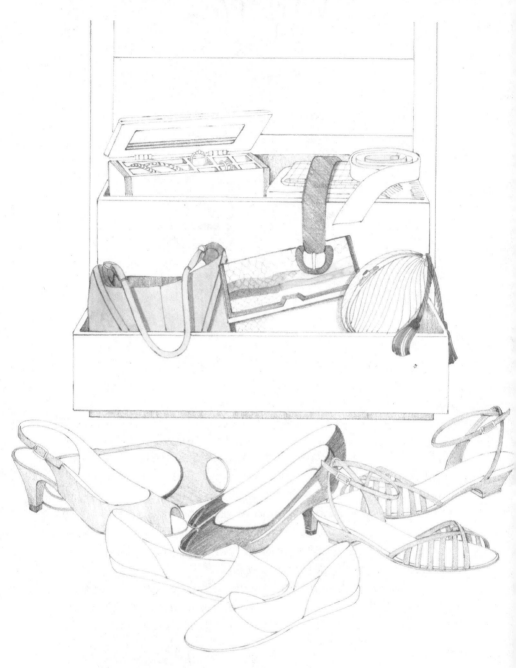

*Accessories are a key ingredient
in putting together your style.*

DAY 8

Developing Your Own Style

tyle is . . . wearing clothes appropriate to your life and to each occasion with ease and comfort.

Style is not . . . simply wearing designer clothing pictured in magazines.

Style is . . . elegance, and that can mean well-cut jeans and a cotton sweater as easily as a smart Italian suit.

Style is not . . . the look singled out by a fashion editor, worn faithfully by the masses.

Style means wearing clothes that look right on you, that feel right and aren't given a second thought during the day. The way they are worn, not the clothes themselves, reflects your style, your attitude, and your way of thinking.

Defining Your Style Profile

How would you characterize yourself? Hectic professional? Down-home casual? Exciting, alive at night? Active, vital, always on-the-go? Your clothes should reflect your lifestyle, and your wardrobe should cater to it: fashion that suits your daily needs.

For the professional, a working wardrobe should take up the most space in your closet. For the city worker, more tailored clothes are needed: suits and silk dresses for the executive; more fashiony, expressive separates for a career in the arts. In the country, more casual clothes work: tweed blazers and gabardine trousers for the professor; silk blouses and dirndl skirts for the doctor.

For the homemaker, a polished variety of activewear separates with a few important dresses or pant and sweater outfits work in both the city and country.

At night, a sequined top and silk pants take you on the town; change sequins for a cashmere sweater for less gala occasions for which you still want to look smart.

On the weekends, the "casualwear" of shetland sweaters and trousers or "fashionwear" of designer sweats offer variation and are appropriate for every woman as long as they suit the occasion.

Every clothing look has its own special style—the couture suit with its detailed design is no more stylish than a pair of red cotton trousers and a matching cotton knit sweater if both have polish and dash and are appropriate. The suit belongs at a board meeting; the red cottons are for picking apples: reverse the two situations and the style is gone. But wear each at the right time and place and you display a keen fashion sense.

What does it take to develop your own style? It involves knowing the look you want to project, the look you will feel at ease with. Example: sexy works only if you live it—constantly checking cleavage and holding closed the sides of a slit skirt won't do it. Better to dress "sophisticated" in more discreet attire. And bear in mind that discreet needn't mean dull: try a V-neck sweater, for instance, instead of a bowtie blouse, with a suit.

Developing your style involves experimenting. An entire day spent at your favorite (or, even better, a previously unexplored) store, trying on a wide range of clothes, including styles you never before thought of wearing. Unlocking the tried-and-true (and boring) pattern is the must-take step. Remember that no one has to see you in any of the clothes; it's just you and the dressing room mirror, so don't be timid. Note: the more expensive departments have larger, more comfortable dressing rooms; try on here, even if you can't buy here. Use the space to walk around in new styles and see how the clothes look on you. Make a list of the ones you like best and find their less expensive counterparts in the moderate-price areas.

Developing your style involves thought. Especially when it calls for spending money. To avoid impulse buying (whose net effect is a closet full of clothes that never get worn), I've devised a strategy; it takes a little longer, but is well worth it. Each season, as I shop the stores looking for new clothes, I start by very quickly going through the various departments I enjoy, rarely stopping to try anything on. Over the next day or two, I recall the best looking items, the most practical ones that will work with pieces I've already got, the few trendy or "fashion statement" items I want for their pizzazz value. I draw up a list and go back to try them on. At second viewing, some of the clothes get crossed off the list before making it to the dressing room. Others die a quick death in there. What I am left with are a few choice items that cover all my fashion bases for that particular time of year.

Developing your style involves trial and error, too. Sometimes you will make a mistake and buy something that, as the saying goes, just isn't you. But turned around, recognizing (even too late) that one look is wrong, and that another is right, means that your fashion persona is evolving, that you are getting closer to that elusive quality known as style. The point here, as always, is to try.

The Elements of Style

Quality

Buy the finest you can afford: natural fabrics, the fullest cuts, the best tailoring. Consider, for example, a black V-neck sweater. If you quickly look at one that costs $15 and another at

$50, you may not see any difference. But take a second, longer look. The more expensive sweater is probably cotton or wool, not synthetic; it will last longer and look better as the years pass. The cheaper sweater will lose its shape faster, pill faster and be hidden in the back of the closet faster, too. Take notice of detailing: the more expensive sweater has the better styling, more contour at the waistline, more interest at the neckline. Spending extra money up front saves time and money in the long run: clothing won't have to be replaced as often.

Quality is reflected in the price tag. But just because an item is expensive doesn't mean you shouldn't still look closely to be sure the price is justified by more than the designer's name. Guard against loose threads and poor seams: quality workmanship is a must.

If you can't afford the better item now, wait for sales. Get in the habit of checking for markdowns. Keep in mind that merchandise slated for a Monday sale is usually put on display the preceding Saturday (late afternoon).

Polyester: fact and fiction

Polyester got its bad rep from those pull-on pants (you know, the ones that cost $9.99 before the markdown!) that molded unflatteringly to every figure flaw. Though not every pair came in that horrid lime-colored waffle design, none were too pretty. Fortunately, not every polyester blend feels like sandpaper nor shines like plastic wrap. Some do indeed feel like silk. If you are very budget conscious and can't afford the real thing, shop carefully to find the best imitation.

Simplicity

The more ornate or fussy a fashion look, the less chance you have of carrying it off with panache. This is as true of multithousand dollar designer creations as of bargain store items, as true of dress styles as of shoe styles. Fashion must always add to your mystique; it must never become center stage, the inevitable end result if you let yourself become a slave to your wardrobe, if you follow every last trend.

Simplicity is often sedate, but not plain or boring. There is nothing plain or boring about a bright red sweater dress. Red is a vibrant color; sweater dressing is alluring. Yet because the color is solid red and the design is one long line, it is simple and stylish. If it had rows of ruffles or a large bull's eye pattern, the element of simplicity would be gone: it would come off as busy and loud.

Fit

Crucial. If the fabric of a garment doesn't drape or lie properly against your body, the item will look as though it were pinned on you, and will feel ghastly.

Fit (and all other criteria) becomes even more important if you are overweight, even a mere five pounds. If a garment is too tight, you'll be uncomfortable in it and your body language will destroy any fashion sense you tried to display (not to mention the risk you run of busting seams and breaking zippers). Buy the size that looks best on you. Don't get hung up on the number: that you can squeeze into a size ten means nothing if it is the fourteen that makes you look and feel right.

Color

To keep your clothes from becoming more important than you are, soft, subdued colors and color combinations say "style." Monochromatic separates always work: a pale pink silk blouse and pale pink wool trousers look fabulous. Bold colors work best with neutrals: a cobalt blue sweater over a white linen skirt.

The color of accessories counts, too—accessories must complete an outfit, not finish it off. When you go monochromatic, accessories can be in the same color family or in a sympathetic color. For the pale pink outfit, add a pink and black patent leather belt and black pumps. When you wear a bold and a neutral, as with the cobalt and white outfit, the accessories must pick up either or both of these colors: cobalt pumps and a white straw purse.

Shopping note: when buying separates, especially in bold colors, complete the outfit that day; trying to match a lone piece on a later shopping expedition rarely works unless you have the piece in hand.

THE ONE AND ONLY BASIC COLOR CHART YOU'LL EVER NEED FOR COLOR COMBINING

sympathetic mixes

white and any other
   single color
     note: the brighter
     the color, the
     chalkier the white
   example: chalk white with cobalt bone
     with teal

black and any other single
   bright or
   neutral except dark,
   murky shades
   (such as brown, green,
   navy, rust)

navy and bone

soft pink and gray

beige and forest green

plum and cream

simply pathetic mixes

navy and red (too cute)

maroon and brown (too
   murky)

teal and orange

beige and brown

gray and brown or
   maroon

kelly green and pink or
   yellow

yellow and brown

mustard and ochre or
   olive drab (in fact,
   avoid these
   colors altogether!)

Fabric

Choosing quality fabrics is part one. Part two is developing a critical eye to pair separates of different fabrics. Rich fabrics (velvet, fine wool, suede, leather) need to be teamed with clothes of equally rich texture—silk blouses, cashmere, angora, or silk blend wool sweaters.

Lighter fabrics are more difficult to judge. *Examples:* A cotton shirt with enough texture to compliment gabardine trousers will be too heavy for cotton-gauze pants. A cable-stitch cotton sweater has enough substance for a thin wool skirt, but not enough for suede—and too much for a thin cotton skirt. A thin cotton knit top would go with the cotton skirt or a pair of mercerized cotton pants. *Conclusion:* Each fabric pairing must be judged individually.

To learn to develop a discriminating eye, get into the habit of feeling the weight and texture of fabrics. Look at the fabric pairings in designer fashion lines to be aware of combination possibilities. Always consider the overall view: how you look in the clothes and how they "move" on you.

Self-interest: the Missing Ingredient

A woman's main fashion problem isn't always undeveloped style or tastes, but rather a lack of interest. If you just don't care, if you pull on whatever's handier at the moment, you simply won't look as great as you can. Even when you're "just running around the corner" for Trixie's cat food, pay attention to yourself.

For all those still saving that beloved, but bedraggled ink-stained shirt from your volunteer days at the community center, or the $40 stone-washed jeans that are now frayed, ripped and stone-dead, throw them out—that is the only way to avoid ever being tempted to wear it again.

If comfort and ease rank highest with you, have a terrific pair of sweats to slip into for those last-minute forays to the market or the laudromat. As Mother always said, you just never know who you'll meet on your way downstairs.

Caring about yourself and about the impression you want to create is part of every aspect of your life. At first thought, dressing might seem a superficial indication, but look again. It is a direct reflection of the way you feel about yourself, from the inside out—never lose sight of this.

25 Fashion Disasters to Avoid at All Costs

1. Knickers with high heels or sandals or anything, except boots.

2. White or bone strappy sandals with a dark evening dress.

3. Dark hose with light shoes.

4. Midcalf boots with anything but pants (worn tucked in or out); with a skirt or dress, they turn your legs chunky and look plain awful!

5. Cuffing jeans with the underside visible. Hem them!!!

6. Jeans with a formal top, especially sequins.

7. Lime anything, anytime, anywhere.

8. Gold clothing during the daytime (includes lamé sneakers).

9. A mix of plaids (and unless you team a bright tartan skirt with a solid sweater, plaids are not too terrifically alluring on a woman).

10. Lots of jewelry in the daytime, especially if you're wearing casual clothes, especially if you're going to the gym!

11. A battle jacket over a dress or suit.

12. A short raincoat with a below-the-knee skirt or dress.

13. Unbelted wrap coats or jackets. If you want to wear the garment open, tie the belt in the back for neatness.

14. Total leather outfits such as a red leather jacket, matching pants, boots and bag. Too much, especially if the leather has a cheap, plasticlike gloss. Pick one leather piece and contrast it

with fine wool. Note: a suede ensemble can work if the garments are made of the very supple, thin suede being manufactured by the better houses.

15. A cheap fur (remember those $200 fur sectionals with each piece dyed a different color?). It's better to wait until you can afford a great fur.

16. A trendy fur piece (example: fur boa with twenty tails) worn over anything but basic black.

17. Wearing more than one trendy garment at a time. Example: your shoulders look great in a slightly padded, asymmetrical collar, white shirt. Terrific, but wear it with the most classic trousers or straight skirt you can find, not a pair of velvet capri pants.

18. Anything so fussy you feel awkward in it. I recently saw a saleswoman at a Fifth Avenue store, who, trying to be very much in vogue, wore a very high-necked ruffled blouse and bib. The look was great, but not on her. She looked completely ill at ease, as though Mother had dressed her up for a fifth grade dance. If it's "not you," forget it.

19. Elasticized-waistband pull-on pants with a polo top tucked in. Too boyish, too cute, too immature. If you like this style of activewear trousers, then jazz it up with a more flattering top: a boat- or scoop-neck T, a pretty hand-knit sweater that covers the elastic waistband, a man-sized shirt to tie on the hips. You know I want you to be comfortable, but alluring, too.

20. Drab dressing. That lifeless attire worn by housewife types on daytime commercials (those that feature bathroom hygiene products in particular). Of course, you mustn't dress up to clean the house, but one gets the idea these women live for their machine washable clothes.

21. The dumpy look: mismatched separates; the hem that is coming undone (you know, the one you try to secure with a few safety pins); the oversized, it-will-hide-the-really-dumpy-clothes-underneath jacket; graceless shoes. Get it together!

22. An oversized shoulder bag at night or with a tailored suit.

23. Artificial flowers clinging to barrettes attached to an un-kempt hairstyle.

24. Hot pink accessories, any season.

25. White patent leather, especially once it has started crack-ing.

SUMMARY OF DAY EIGHT

1. Analyze your lifestyle to determine
the fashion image most appropriate for you.

2. Look for the elements of style when
shopping for clothes: quality; simplicity;
fit; color; fabric.

3. When shopping, learn to evaluate
the usefulness of each item you consider.
Buying might take place another day,
after careful reflection.

Fashion Forum I: Image Dressing for Daytime

A lot of people find fault with the expression clothes make the person. Of course, clothes can't define character, but they certainly do reflect it. When you wake up on Saturday morning and slip into faded jeans and a T-shirt to do your dreaded weekend chores, you tell the world, "I'm feeling slouchy." When you spend an extra half-hour meticulously selecting clothes in preparation for the party you're going to that night, you are saying, "I'm excited about tonight, and I'm going to sparkle." There are no two ways about it: your clothes do speak for you.

And clothes do help make the woman. The right attire certainly gets you the respect and attention you want. That is why daytime dressing is every bit as important as evening clothes. Whether you have a temporary job or a lifelong career, clothes count. Perhaps the element that comes first is pride: pride in whatever work you are doing, and pride in yourself. There is a young woman I know who is a receptionist at an ad agency. She likes her work, but is not at all interested in having a career. Consequently, she pays little attention to what is appropriate office attire, preferring to wear whatever cute outfit strikes her fancy in the morning. In warm weather, she might be wearing turquoise cotton trousers, a Hawaiian print shirt and strappy sandals. In the winter, she'll have on bright leg warmers and an oversized ski sweater. She looks great . . . for a Saturday afternoon, but not for the office, certainly not as the first person a client sees when entering the lobby. This woman lacks a sense of esteem and pride; she considers her job play, not the serious business it is—a representative for the firm. Whether or not her employers accept her "style" is not my first concern: it's getting her to want to change for herself, not just to keep her job (dressing out of demand creates resentment she shouldn't have to feel; dressing out of desire creates the self-image she deserves to feel). If this woman sounds familiar to you, take action—and grow up: take yourself and your work more seriously.

The Business Suit:
Why It Doesn't Work for Most Women

One of the great misfortunes of entering the man's marketplace is having to dress like a man. Suits look great—on men. Suits look like little uniforms on women. If the jacket hides the waist, it's unflattering. If the skirt is cut too straight, it's unflattering. If you must wear a blouse with a cutesy tie or bow (the ultimate defeminizing transposition), it's unflattering. Men look great in ties; women look like they are choking.

Alternatives

If you've been dressing with the primary goal of "blending in," it's time to exert your individuality, not with turquoise trousers exactly, but with one of the many other alternatives.

1. The dress

No, you don't have to top it with a blazer! A simple silk dress stands on its own. For a professional look, choose a style with sleeves (spaghetti straps aren't appropriate for work in most corporate arenas). The sweater dress, the shirtwaist dress and the coatdress with its suitlike styling are other polished dress alternatives—fantastic with accessories.

2. The "cardigan" suit

Knits are always more alluring than stiff polyblends. Knit sweaters, styled like a jacket, give you the suit look without the mannishness. A close-fitting cardigan that buttons like a blouse (and therefore takes the place of one) looks great belted and teamed with a skirt or trousers. Another variation is the three piece knit suit: top, skirt, and cardigan which is worn open for a soft look.

3. The super blouse

A namby-pamby self-tie blouse needs help, it's true. But a stylized blouse, with shoulder padding and an exciting, asymmetrical neckline stands on its own with a slim skirt (if you have slim hips) or trousers. A tuxedo shirt accomplishes the same result—but instead of reaching for the ubiquitous shoestring tie, fasten an antique bar pin at the collar.

4. The unconstructed blazer

If you must wear a jacket, choose this flexible alternative. Push up the sleeves for panache and team it with a V- or boatneck blouse or sweater for style. (Add pearls if you need to feel more establishment.) In a neutral color, like bone or gray, this jacket will work with skirts as well as trousers. As long as you mix solid blocks of color, rather than colors and prints, the look is great. Such a blazer will add professional polish to simple (not to be confused with "super"—see #3) blouses and sweaters.

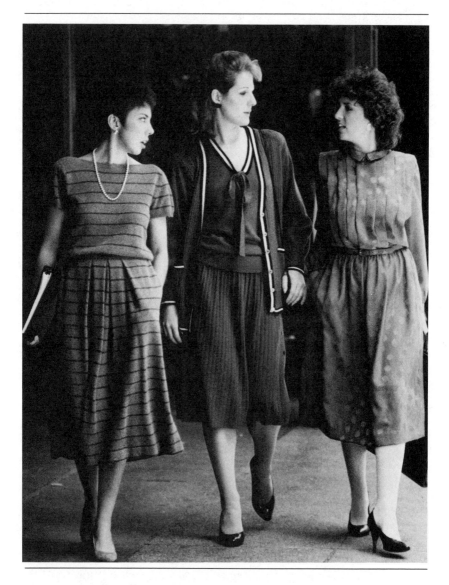

Michele is wearing a two-piece ensemble, a navy-stripe on beige knit. Perfectly pulled together.

Annemarie's three-piece cardigan suit looks great with/ without the oversweater. The solid red skirt unbuttons on the side to reveal a slit for evening wear.

Elaine's sapphire blue silk dress, with its double collar and sophisticated pleating, wears beautifully (without a blazer!).

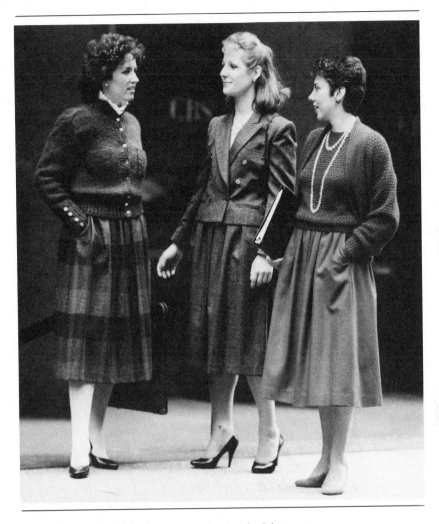

Elaine's emerald tweed sweater jacket teams
with a skirt in a "stained glass" plaid of clear
blues and greens. The super blouse with its ruffled
collar works on its own during warm months.

Annemarie's made-in-America European-styled
suit is a tiny black and white tweed. The close-
fitted waistjacket needs only pearls (not a
shirt) to complete the high-powered look.

Michele's burgundy sweater set, shown here
with a matching wool skirt, would team equally
well with black pleated trousers (and with
a change from the taupe shoes to black ones).

5. The European-tailored suit

What is most objectionable about the typical navy suit is the paper doll cutout look most mass-marketed American suits have. But European tailoring can be quite flattering—a "name" house offers high chic, with a high price tag. These suits (many of which do not require a blouse, thus giving them added pizzazz) are for the very tall and slim and graceful—it takes courage just to try one on. If you must have a suit, this is the one to get. (Note: some American designers, such as Calvin Klein, have brought this high styling to their lines, at much lower prices than true Europeans.)

6. The two-piece ensemble

A matching blouse and skirt, in either a print or solid color, have enough polish to go without a jacket (for warmth, add a stylish solid cardigan). As long as the two pieces coordinate perfectly, and by that I mean "match" (more harmonious and pulled together than contrasting separates), you achieve a total, dress-like look. Don't forget accessories; they add more dash and a bit of individuality.

Clothes on the Go: Casual Doesn't Mean Careless

No matter how slouchy you might feel, resist the temptation to be careless, even on your own time.

Style is twenty-four hours a day. But you say you love play clothes. Great! So do I. Just buy them carefully. Instead of budget sweats, buy Norma Kamali, within nearly everyone's budget yet with such style and flair that you look special. Instead of cheap painter's pants, buy Liz Claiborne or Jones New York activewear. Instead of peasant dresses (you know, the kind made from cotton that looks permanently creased), buy Laura Ashley or Jessica McClintock sundresses. No matter how casual you get, always look for style and quality. Yes, these are often built into the price, but you do get as much as you pay for.

What's in a Label?

Each and every garment was designed by someone—the lowliest T-shirt was created by a fashion designer! A handful of designers have become so popular that they are more than the creative employee at a fashion house: they are the fashion house. Are these the only names that should be on your labels? Not necessarily.

America's top designers do produce a fashion line each season (five or six fashion seasons a year). This pricey collection is the core of their design work. Additionally, they license their name to be used on all sorts of garments and products that they may or may not have designed. The great fallacy in wearing T-shirts with a designer logo or jeans with a designer name is that the designer in question might have had nothing at all to do with designing the item! The best designer clothes are the ones with the labels on the inside—you want to give the impression of having your own style, not just borrowing someone else's. As the slogan for an expensive yet discreet line of leather goods goes, your own initials are enough.

But are the designer clothes so far superior? Most likely, the fabrics are more costly and the handcrafting more elaborate on higher priced goods. And yet the styling itself (which cannot be registered or patented) will not be unique for long. The trickle-down effect is quite present in the fashion industry. A designer blouse complete with chic detailing and a $400 price tag will be slightly simplified by a "better" fashion house and sold for $150. The "moderate" manufacturer will simplify it even further and offer it for $70, and finally, maybe six months to a year later, a "budget" line will offer it for $20. Of course, the blouse is not exactly the same, but the basic shape or look will be saved. Depending on your budget, and how long the style will be correct, you will choose accordingly.

There is a label in every item of clothing offered for sale—

you have the right to know where and by whom it was made. How much importance that label has for you is a personal decision. More critical considerations are how the garment looks on you, how it fits into your lifestyle, and, very simply, how much you like it. One rule to follow: don't be so hung up on labels that you keep yourself from discovering new and talented designers often featured only at small shops. Never let fashion stop being fun.

SUMMARY OF DAY NINE

1. Recognize that clothes are a strong reflection of your personality. The way you dress at work tells others how dedicated and concerned you are.

2. Don't limit yourself to the standard suit. You can be an individual and still be appropriately dressed. Consider the six fashion alternatives to the blue serge cookie-cutter look.

3. Maintain your fashion sense during private time as well. Casual should never be careless.

4. Familiarize yourself with the styles of top designers, then find other fashion houses who translate their looks into more budget-conscious fashions. Investigate young, new designers who showcase in smaller boutiques or special areas within a department store.

Fashion Forum II: Image Dressing for Nighttime

Thumbing through the pages of *Vogue* and *Harper's Bazaar*, one gets the impression that a decent evening gown costs about $4,000. "Guess we'll be staying home tonight . . ." you murmur. Not necessarily . . .

Getting Past Lime Organza

Not in organza, nor chiffon, not even in silk is this a color to be worn, especially after dark. The only place to have lime in your life is in your club soda. Black is the color of the night, followed by gold, and then white. If you have a pair of black silk pants or a black slip dress, you can go anywhere and be captivating. There might be a thousand women at a formal occasion, but if you are wearing a one-shoulder black gown, you will be the one noticed. For even the most casual dresser, black works: wear a soft, deep V'd black sweater and push the sleeves up to the elbows—undeniably sexy, over white trousers or even jeans.

Simplicity, one of the watchwords of style, is a nonnegotiable rule at night. Pare down to the simplest pieces. The more paraphernalia you have on, the less elegant the look. Gold coin earrings, marabou boas, and snake bracelets connote carnival, not allure. It's the difference between looking glamorous and looking garish. Also, classic, pared-down styles are sexier, and make you more approachable. A taffeta designer dress with its flamboyant neck and sleeve treatment might look stunning in a magazine, but the dress keeps *you* from being noticed: like a barricade, it stands between you and other people—fine if you are a presenter at the next Oscars awards ceremony, not so fine if you are anywhere else.

Here is a rundown of evening options to collect:

- Black silk pants or, if you are too hippy, a black silk skirt, to be teamed with one of the options below.
- A silk camisole; these are available in every size, and can be worn by every woman. If you are too endowed to go without a bra, buy yourself a well-fitted strapless bra or, even better, a bustier which is fitted to the waist for comfort and complete control. Naturally, a black camisole will be very dramatic, but you can wear any bold color with a black skirt or pants.
- A beaded black sweater for colder months (the silk pants can be worn year-round). Again, you might choose a sweater in another color, but going monochromatic at night works best.
- A black dress: a silk slip style if you are thin, a wrap style if you are not. A slightly mini (just above the knee) sweater dress, belted with a thin black lizard belt and worn with black patent leather pumps is a knockout, too.

Once you have the basics, you may repeat the two-piece top and pants/skirt outfit in another color: red silk pants and a red beaded top; a plum silk skirt and a plum angora sweater. Bright

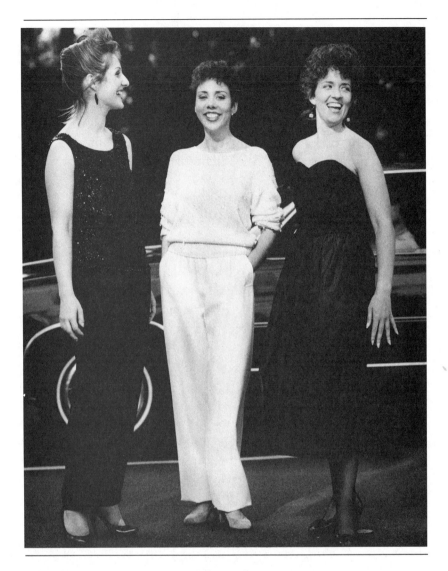

Annemarie is dazzling in a black sequin-and-bead top and straight-leg black silk pants.

Michele is wearing a fabulous white sweater adorned with clear drops and white trousers. (A white wool slit skirt would be terrific, too).

Elaine is total glamor in this strapless dress with a velvet bodice and taffeta skirt. Note: this look belongs only in black; switch the color and the drama disappears.

colors can work as long as you keep the one-color rule for evening.

Note: the one great advantage to black is that the color conceals otherwise obvious signs of cheapness, hence you can look stunning in a very inexpensive pair of black silk pants (silks vary—you can buy pants at $40 or $400!). However, when you start wearing other colors, quality becomes much more important and increases as the color lightens; wear white only when you can afford the best.

Accessories: Make It or Break It

The accessories you wear with your clothes are as important as the clothes themselves. And when you are on a limited budget, a variety of accessories can make the same sweater dress look different, even if you wear it twice a week. Because daytime clothes tend to be more tailored, carrying a large shoulderbag or wearing what Grandmother would call sensible shoes is accepted. But the skimmed look of night attire demands pared-down accessories.

With black pants, black pumps (very useful daytime, too) are the perfect choice. They work with a sleeved dress, too. But if you are wearing a slip dress or a camisole or anything strapless, the bareness at your neck and shoulders needs to be complemented by open shoes: sling backs or strappy sandals, both with a medium to high heel, and in black. Silver, gold and other metallics are not as sophisticated nor as chic as you have been led to believe. If you are being daring and are wearing one of these colors overall, be sure the matching shoes are of dyed leather, not plastic, for the richest effect.

Your purse must be equally pared down at night. A small clutch, a gold or gold-toned maudinière (a small boxy or oval metal case on a thin chain, fitting in the palm of your hand), or a slim shoulderbag, no more than 7" long, are delicate choices, big enough to hold lipstick, keys, money (you really don't need to lug your five-year calendar-planner to dinner!).

Most dressy evening tops won't need a belt, but some other fashions might benefit from this finishing touch. An excellent choice is a 2″ wide length of satin ribbon, available in every color imaginable at a notions store. A thin gold belt, a thin black lizard belt, or satin cord (also available at the notions store) are other great options that are downright inexpensive and very adaptable.

Jewelry is a sensual touch nearly every woman loves. And how right it is at night. Yet it is usually an either/or choice because too much is wrong. If you have a very dramatic piece, such as a nine-strand beaded necklace or a very wide ivory bracelet, it deserves center stage; other items, such as earrings and rings, must be very simple. I like thin, dangling earrings. Because they come close to the shoulders, I don't wear a necklace with them. If instead I want to wear a few of my gold hearts (from a collection started before I fell in love with thin, dangling earrings), I'll wear plain gold studs or very small hoops in my ears. Either one or the other, but not both.

Gold jewelry—and less expensive art jewelry being created in bronze and gold-over-bronze—is great, perfect for night. So are pearls and, if you've saved your money, diamonds. While fun jewelry made of wood, other metals, and even the new, high gloss plastics are inexpensive accoutrements for day, they are not right at night—better to go bare (that can be just as alluring).

What you wear over your "night clothes" counts, too. A raincoat just won't make it. Invest in an oversized shawl that works like a light cape—again in black, it will always look right, even by day. "But I won't wear it that often," you think to yourself. Ah, but yes you will: once you have one, you'll see just how versatile it is and will find yourself reaching for it quite often.

In cold weather, a heavier wool cape is the choice. It can also function as a daytime coat, as easily over pants as a dress.

The ultimate is a fur. There is nothing like it. I'm not talking about that $99 rabbit section battle jacket now. I'm talking pelts! Yes, it is an investment of at least $3,000 and could be twice that (or more). But the feeling of luxury and, frankly, of power that a woman feels wrapped in a coat or lush jacket is immeasurable. Flexible payment plans make it easier than you think to own one, but only if you are ready to pay for quality. If not, buy yourself the most wonderful wool coat you can find.

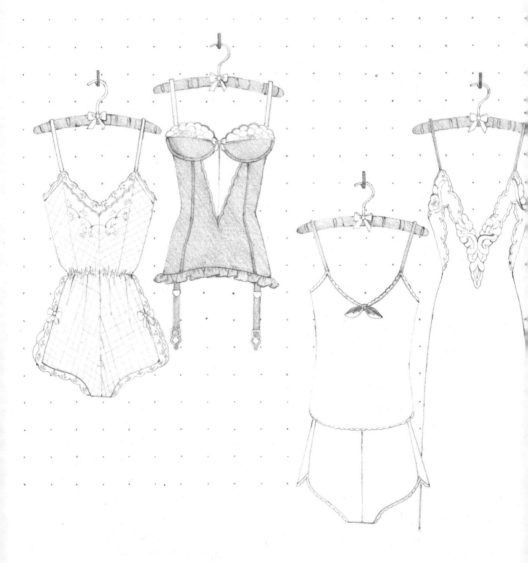

The very beginnings of a collection.

Your Evening Persona: Is Every Woman Sexy?

If you look up "sexy" in *Webster's*, you'll find the unhelpful description, "sexually suggestive." If you look up "sexual," you'll find "relating to, or associated with sex." And if you look up "sex," you'll find "sexually motivated behavior." Talk about getting the runaround! But the truth is, sexy is in the eye of the beholder. And quite hard to define. It is a feeling that comes from within, an attitude you project with your entire being. Put a woman in the skimpiest bikini and she still won't look sexy unless she exudes it. And by the same token, if you change her into a crewneck sweater and a demure strand of pearls, she can appear almost sensual, if she projects the attitude.

Every woman has the potential to look sexy (just as every man does). And why shouldn't she? There is nothing unfeminist about being feminine, about putting forth the effort to be alluring, especially if she does it to feel good about herself. The best part is, sexy means whatever you want it to mean and takes whatever form you want it to take. All that matters is that you feel natural. "Sexy" is not a lure to catch a man or wrangle a job. It is a state of mind that tells you that you have appeal and confidence, that gets you feeling good about yourself and eager to try for things you never let yourself dream about before. Being sexy is, if nothing else, the opposite of being afraid.

Boudoir Basics: Allure in the Bedroom

Want to know a big secret? Men love lingerie. They love teddies, and camisoles, and tap pants, and corselettes, and stockings, and some of them even like those marabou-trimmed slippers! And why shouldn't they? These underpinnings are gorgeous. And flattering. Is there anything wrong in looking gorgeous for the man in your life? No. Especially not if you request the same of him.

If you've never browsed through the foundations department at a neighborhood store, you might feel a bit timid. Don't. The saleswomen are very familiar with the popularity of these lacy confections and, once given your measurements, will help you, no disapproving look or snide smile about it.

Many lingerie catalogues let you shop in the privacy of your own boudoir (they advertise in all the right magazines, too); just be certain of your sizes because much of the merchandise is not returnable.

Sweet dreams.

SUMMARY OF DAY TEN

1. At night, simplicity is the rule: stark colors (black is best), pared-down designs.

2. Black pants, with an appropriate top, or a black knee-length dress will take you anywhere.

3. Watch accessories: again, simple and pared-down to avoid cluttering the bare lines of your clothing.

The Impact of Perfume

F act: we are each aroused by scent. Ever since Cleopatra scented the sails on her barge to announce her arrival to Marc Antony, women have been using fragrance to add to their allure, to send a special message.

Perfume is a habit to be developed. Yet because it can be so distracting, it must be used carefully. A light scent or lighter concentration (eau de toilette or cologne) of a richer fragrance adds a note of polish for day wear without seeming unprofessional. At night, when you want to mesmerize, a more complex fragrance or the heavier perfume concentration of your favorite scent is appropriate.

How to Shop for a Fragrance

The staggering number of fragrances on the market can make selecting one a dizzying experience (second only to buying

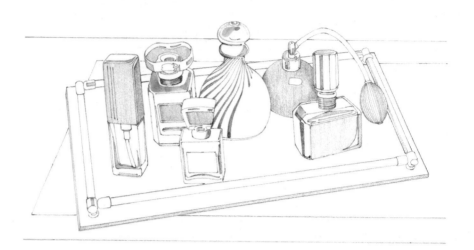

makeup!). You won't find your scent on your first try—and don't try to. A perfume can become your signature, a very strong identification—selecting something this important should take time, and should be treated as an adventure.

You may combine a perfume expedition with a shopping trip. When you reach the store, head to the fragrance counter first. The testers (open bottles of each fragrance) will help you narrow the choices. Start by spraying one in the air, about six inches from your nose. This is to tell if the scent appeals to you. Repeat this test with other fragrances until you have selected two you want to try on your skin.

Spray one of the scents on your right forearm, the other on the left. Ask yourself if you still like either. Perfume will smell a bit different on you than in the air as it mixes with your skin's own chemistry. What you are inhaling now are the top notes, the first layer of the scent. Within the hour, the middle notes will emerge, altering your perception of the fragrance. In two or more hours, the base, or final layer of the perfume, develops— this is the longest lasting of the three. It is important to sense all these notes to determine whether or not you like the full range of each scent you try. As you shop, periodically inhale the two scents you are wearing. Do this after thirty minutes, one hour, two hours and three hours.

If, at the end of your shopping, you like either (or both!) scents, buy a small flacon of either the perfume, cologne, or eau de toilette strengths (perfume, which contains more oils, less alcohol, than the other two, last longer, goes further, and costs more). Resist buying the larger sizes despite the overall savings reflected in the full ounce bottles because you may not stay fond of any one scent as you actually start wearing it.

If neither scent appeals to you at the end of the day, try to locate samples of other scents. Ask a salesperson behind the fragrance counter if the store has any trial sizes to give away to customers. There are always special promotions going on to introduce new perfumes—look for company reps or the sales staff strolling through the main floor with baskets of samples. Take these home to try another day. Don't spray any other scents on your arms while still in the store, even if you no longer smell the first two—traces will remain until you shower or bathe and will confuse your nose.

To continue your search for the perfect scent, in addition to using the testers every time you are in a department store, check the following:

- bill enclosures featuring scented cards; rub the card right on your wrist to get a better idea of the scent;
- magazine inserts marked "scratch and sniff" or the newer folder cards you snap open to reveal the scent; again rub the paper on your wrist;
- department store mailings that announce a new perfume and invite you to stop in for a sample;

Why all the effort over finding a scent? Because it offers you an added dimension of appeal. Because a scent will blend with you and smell differently on you than on every other woman, thereby distinguishing you. Because everyone is attracted by a provocative aroma: just as your looks attract others, so does your personal scent. Perfume creates an impression: aside from making you feel special when you put it on, it tells the world how you feel about yourself.

The one reason not to choose a particular scent: because it smells terrific on someone else. That has to do with *her* body chemistry, with the way the oils and flavors in the perfume mix with *her* skin. Yes, it is wonderful that every fragrance will smell special on each woman who wears it, but the flip side means that you can only be sure of how it will smell on you only after you try it and wait for it to "bloom."

Perfume: Art and Science

Perfume will be forever likened to a musical composition (a symphony to boot) because each and every fragrance is a blend of dozens of different individual scents: essential oils extracted from flowers, herbs and spices, and even fruits! Depending on the balance of the ingredients, a fragrance can be classified as a floral (with notes of rose, jasmine, muguet, hyacinth, violet to name a few); a spice (cinnamon, nutmeg, vanilla, cloves, pepper, sage aren't for the kitchen only); or a citrus (not just orange and lemon, but actually any fruit might be in the newer combinations). Though the art of blending a popular fragrance does involve a bit of science, you needn't get too technical. Because the only question that really needs an answer is: do you like the way it smells and do others compliment you on it?

The Dimensions of Fragrance

Just as a fragrance is composed of many layers, so can you increase its dimensions by using a variety of scented products (of the same perfume) and by scenting your clothes as well.

Yes, this is an indulgence, one every woman should experience:

- the pleasure of pouring a capful of perfumed cleansing gel on a loofah sponge and invigorating your skin;
- the gentleness of smoothing on scented body lotion (before toweling off to preserve moisture);
- the dusting on of scented talc with a soft, large puff;
- the splash of cologne;
- slipping into clothes that have picked up just the slightest bit of scent from perfume-doused sachets;
- and finally, dabbing perfume at the pulse points and anywhere your imagination takes you.

Notice the positive reaction of others: the impact is unmistakable, well worth the effort.

```
┌───────────────SUMMARY OF DAY ELEVEN───────────────┐
│                                                    │
│  1. Make perfume part of your daily ritual. Take   │
│  the time to make it a habit; it's one you will    │
│  enjoy.                                            │
│                                                    │
│  2. Continually investigate new fragrances until   │
│  you find the one that becomes your signature.     │
│                                                    │
│  3. Layer fragrance by using companion products    │
│  and scenting clothes, linens, even light          │
│  bulbs (whose heat radiates the scent).            │
│                                                    │
└────────────────────────────────────────────────────┘
```

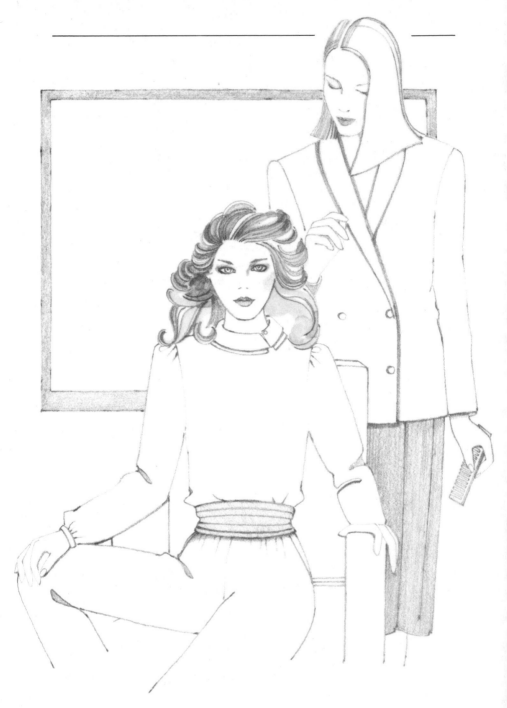

A fabulous look is the result of a skilled
stylist, and the rapport the two of you share.

DAY 12

Hairstyle:
an Essential Fashion

Surprised to find a chapter on hair in the style section rather than in beauty? Surprise! Your hair has a crucial role to play in the stylish image you create. Having healthy, shiny, manageable hair is a must, but there is more. Your hair is a great personality indicator. Picture Goldie Hawn's mass of long waves: it shouts gregarious; Linda Evans' subdued, almost demure coiffure: it whispers sensuality; and Olivia Newton-John's short, sexy cut: it looks alive, perky.

Why do all three hair images work equally well? Because each was designed for the individual face, lifestyle and image. In the quest for finding the right look, American women devote more time, energy and money to hair than to makeup. Unfortunately, much of that time is wasted. Why? They try to effect the change themselves instead of trusting in a skilled hairstylist to work the techniques that will enhance. Yes, you can improve the quality of your hair (follow the same guidelines that apply to improving skin quality and allover good health, listed on page

51), but to improve its character through color, texture, and shape, you need a professional.

The essence of this chapter is to clue you into the image changes you can achieve by changing your hairstyle, not to add to the mountain of books on hair coloring, hair perming, and hair styling that are virtually pointless because you simply cannot achieve the promised results at home.

Choosing a Stylist

The unbendable rule of hair beauty and style: find a stylist who understands your hair needs and to whom you feel comfortable talking. Popular theory likens the relationship of a woman and her hairdresser to that of a man and his bartender: friend, confidant, soulmate. It is true. Women feel very protective of their hair; it is an important, outward sign of femininity. To let someone get that close, to literally place this treasure in another person's hands, breaks down most of the barriers we are able to set up with others. If you don't feel a kinship with your hairdresser, the awkwardness of having him or her this close can be unbearable, and the results, disastrous. How to find the right hairdresser? Again, it involves crossing boundaries, being vocal about your desires, asserting yourself to get what you want, the overall objective.

1. Discovery

There are basically three types of hair salons: the "name" salon, built around the reputation of one key stylist (José Eber, Vidal Sassoon, Kenneth) with other hand-picked and well-trained stylists; the fashion store salon (Saks Fifth Avenue, Lord & Taylor); the neighborhood beauty parlor. The differences: price, those above being listed in descending order; technique, the name salon offering the most avant-garde styles, fashion oriented and often too severe; availability and rapport, with the neighborhood shop often being the most willing to accommodate you.

2. Evaluation

What do you want from the salon you choose? High drama is built into the look of the name stylist—you are his/her walking advertisement; the more processes you want, the more technique-experienced you want your stylist to be. A style of simplicity and easy care might be better achieved at the local salon, and the lower cost might mean you can go there for styling two or three times for every trim or touch-up visit at the others—great if you are all thumbs at home or simply like to feel pampered before a big day or night. The fashion store salon offers convenience and perhaps more ingenuity than the neighborhood place, at a price more reasonable than the name stylist.

Once you know what your needs are, it is time to evaluate the options. Regardless of the type of salon you choose, make a list of three possibilities (even among the neighborhood shops, there is some degree of difference). Investigate each one: examine the photos the shop displays and ask which stylist is responsible for each cut; ask to speak to the stylist whose work you like, even if this means making an appointment for a consultation; explain your needs and your desires and gauge his/her response: accommodating? brusque? full of suggestions? Then make a first impression assessment: do you feel comfortable, or anxious? does he/she inspire confidence? (Your role here is the key: if you don't express yourself honestly, the stylist can't serve you adequately.)

Visits to a few establishments might be necessary before you find one that satisfies you. Be selective. Do not feel obligated because you took up a few minutes of a stylist's time—if it makes you more comfortable, or if the stylist requests it, pay a nominal fee or a gratuity for the time given you. But do not allow anyone you have doubts about to cut your hair.

3. The tryout

The best way to judge a stylist's work is to see him/her in action. However, you don't need to be a sacrificial lamb. For the first appointment, limit the treatment to a shampoo and styling or a trim—just enough to add shape and dimension without making a drastic change. Engage the stylist in conversation. Discuss the processes to be considered for your next visit: a more dramatic cut, highlighting, a perm/body wave or straightening. Ask questions that have been bothering you—perhaps that nagging dry scalp condition, or hair breakage (actually, a top stylist will point these out to you and suggest treatment at home and, if necessary, at the salon). Don't worry about becoming chums overnight: the relationship will develop on its own. But do speak up if you want to establish a good working rapport. Your stylist deserves to be treated as a person, not a servant. Though you might be silent out of fear or innocence, he/she might misinterpret your coldness as arrogance, and that's no way to begin a long-term association.

Once you find a stylist you want to work with, treasure the relationship. The better the stylist knows you, the better he/she can treat your hair.

4. Finding your look

If you're like me, you arrive for a haircut armed with a multitude of magazine clippings showing hairstyles. These are useful to convey the general shape of the cut you want. Additionally, you and your stylist should discuss how to adapt a particular style to the shape of your face and the quality of your hair, to make the look more yours. The style you select should be one you can easily maintain. If it requires a curling iron or electric rollers, be sure the stylist shows you how to use them. And ask yourself if you have the time to use them. If your daily schedule is booked up as it is, ask about getting a perm or body wave for wash-dry-and-go hair that needs just a bit of finger work to fall into place. Unless you can afford twice-a-week visits to your stylist for settings, a dramatic in-salon look will be worthless if you can't duplicate it at home.

Some women arrive at their salon knowing they want a change, but haven't a strong idea of what the specifics ought to be. In this case, let your stylist's creativity go to work. Offer some clues (dramatic/carefree/casual) and then listen to his/her ideas. By manipulating your hair, he/she can give you an idea of how the finished cut will look. By paying attention, you will sense if the style is too extreme or just the switch you are looking for. Note: a stylist you know well and have been working with for some time can be trusted to give you what you want; the name stylist who is a stranger to you, but who you've been dying to see (and have been saving up for) may not give you the results you'd expect.

The Impact of a Hat: A Dramatic Alternative

It takes a lot of self-confidence to wear a hat. To those who have never thought of adding this accessory to their wardrobe, the first time you try one on can seem as awkward as balancing a book on your head. What great women of style know, however, is that the drama that accompanies the wearing of a great hat (I'm not talking demure pillbox here!) is fantastic and alluring.

The easiest way to explore hat wearing is in the warm weather months. For $20, you can have a most exquisite wide-brimmed straw hat—one which goes as well with a sundress as with a bright white suit or a linen trouser-and-blouse pairing. Using one or two large hat pins will secure it: no need to walk with one hand on your head! The way in which a hat shades your eyes is very provocative and creates a mystique: people just can't help wanting to see exactly what's under that brim.

If you find you like the straw hat, try another, perhaps a brightly lacquered one in red or black. In cooler months, colored straw gives way to a lush felt fedora. In winter, a knit cap trimmed with a wide band of fur frames the face in appealing softness.

The one requisite to wearing a hat: you must wear the simplest hairstyle possible, such as a chignon at the nape of the neck, or one that is loose and straight to look sleek, not "deflated," should you take the hat off.

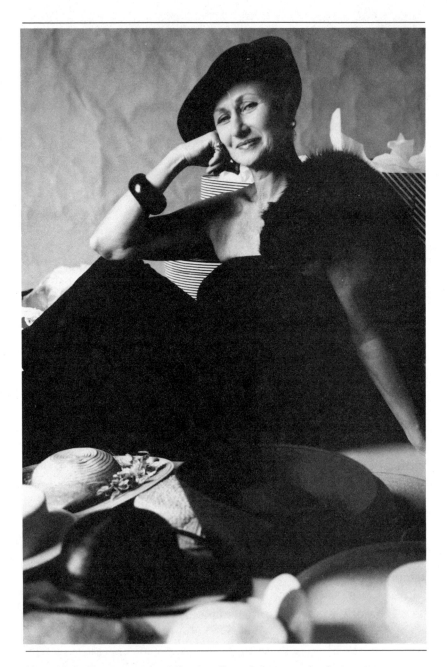

New York literary agent Roslyn Targ is known for her hats. She is pictured with only part (!) of her collection and another treasured accessory, a lush black fox boa appropriately nicknamed Spellbinder.

1. Make finding a skilled stylist a priority.
The search will take time and involves footwork and
thought, but the energy spent will be nominal
considering a stylist can be yours for life.

2. Before insisting on a certain style, evaluate
its practicality in your life. Consider maintenance
costs and at-home attention. A simple cut can look
as classic and stylish as the most extravagant one,
more so if your upkeep abilities aren't strong enough
to recreate the extravagant style on your own.

3. Be daring and experiment with a dramatic hat—
aside from the fashion advantages, you'll save
yourself considerable hairstyling time.

DAY 13

Lifestyle:
Easy Surroundings

tyle is not just a fashion image; it is a way of life, an ease with which you move from one occasion to another. Just as you feel at ease with your clothes when you know they look and wear well (think of the dis-ease you feel when you've tacked up a loose hem with tape or replaced a button with a safety pin), so should you be at ease with your surroundings by making your home a comfortable place to be.

That sounds like common sense and yet how many times have you had guests over and felt uneasy or somewhat less than a perfect hostess? The main reason for social paranoia is awkwardness born of discomfort. Example: you spend a fortune to have your living room properly furnished—it's so lovely you're nervous about sitting on the sofa. Well, that uneasiness transfers to your guests, spoiling a party.

Some people are comfortable with crystal and silver; others think they should have these things, yet aren't really at home with them because of fears of breakage or tarnishing. If you'd feel "safer" with stainless steel, that's what you should have—for good looks, those with brightly colored handles are terrific. What works best is what works best for you.

If you're wondering what utensils have to do with style, the answer is everything. The way you decorate your home and your office, the way you set a table, the flowers you choose for the vase on your desk or to send to a new acquaintance: these are all ways in which you communicate your style sense. The point, then, is to make your style not just something you put on in the morning, but an attitude you live and breathe every day.

Home Style

Your home, whether a house or an apartment, should be a haven you look forward to returning to after work, a special place which you can share with friends, a place that reflects you. You don't need a decorator and a $10,000 budget to accomplish this. You need a sense of self. For that, sit down with paper and pencil and decide on what would make your home more perfect. Is it matching table settings for those intimate dinner parties you'd love to give? Is it the homey feeling that comes from large throw pillows scattered on the rug and on your bed? Is it a touch of glamor—a large red paper fan hung as art? The right answer is the one that pleases you.

Many women know what they want—price tags are what keep them from obtaining the must haves. But with creativity, a skimpy budget can appear to be stretched.

Start with a color scheme. Repeat your best fashion colors at home. Mix two or three bold colors or up to five shades of a single color family for richness and harmony.

Build-it-yourself basics are inexpensive and quickly available. Paint wood platforms to match or coordinate with wall color and dress with cushions and pillows in the closest possible shade. Stripping wood floors and shining them with polyurethane means skipping a rug. If living area windows offer a great view, take down blinds and forget drapes.

Just as accessories make up for a limited wardrobe, use home furnishings to complete your home style. Frame $5 and $10 posters for the look of expensive prints. Buy oversized glass or ceramic vases and fill with dried flowers (spray with your perfume for a seductive touch). Drape a lace shawl over your bed in between wearings. Turn two large scarves into a throw pillow. Cover the entire top of an end table with your pill box or frog collection—display things that mean something to you.

Work in stages—few people complete their decorating in one swoop. Wait until you can afford the pieces you really want rather than wasting money on transitional items you'll end up hating. Devise a tentative schedule for acquiring your worldly possessions and watch how quickly your dreams take shape.

Entertaining Style

I've always thought that women starting out on a new career and a new home after completing their education should be given the same kind of shower traditionally reserved for brides. (Single women tend to do even more entertaining than couples!)

A great advantage to setting up house on one's own is being able to choose exactly what you want. Start by deciding on your look—casual or formal, country or dramatic. Do you want linen napkins and matching quilted placemats or will paper napkins over straw mats do as nicely? Must you have glasses for water, wine, and soft drinks or will an all-purpose bowl-shaped glass do for all three (yes!)? Your serving pieces and tableware should naturally reflect your fashion and furnishings style.

Then take an inventory of what you have. Get rid of those seven mismatched glasses and buy a set of six or eight, once and for all (restaurant supply stores have great discounts on quality merchandise—the first stop on your shopping expedition). Browse for the china and table linens you'd like to have. Buy one or two place settings at a time and, if you are very conscious of everything being "just so," invite over only as many people as

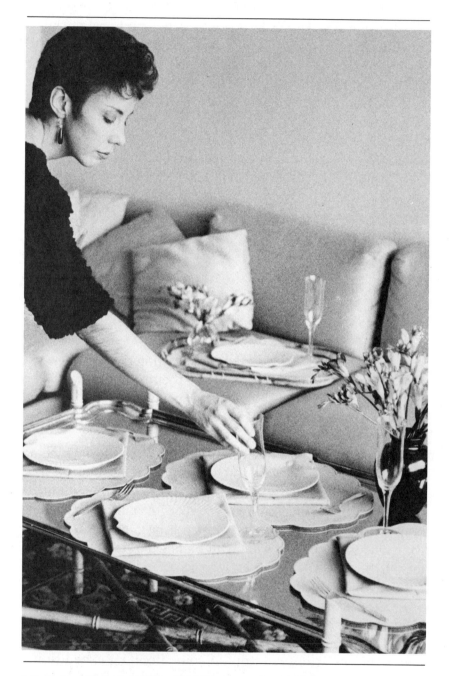

Michele sets her coffee table for dinner; bamboo
trays repeat the place settings, right down to bud
vases, when entertaining more than four.

you have settings for. (A dinner party for three now gives you the confidence you'll need to entertain eight later.)

Think of your guests' comfort as well as your own. With today's smaller apartments, dining rooms are rare—even an alcove is hard to come by! Savvy hostesses know they can serve around a large coffee table. And with inexpensive wicker trays, dinner can be eaten anywhere, and with great panache.

Little touches are very important, and much appreciated: small vases of little flowers add festivity; a brightly colored, fluffy hand towel and a scented guest-size medallion of soap in the bath; a well-made bed for coats if there isn't enough closet space; soft lighting to create a relaxed atmosphere (and flattering glow).

To prevent last-minute trips to the grocery, not to mention hostess panic, make up a schedule the day before a party. Have a master shopping list written as well as a third sheet detailing the serving pieces needed for each dish. Working up lists might seem like extra work, but this organization provides you with a sense of assurance and that keeps you calm and confident.

Office Style

As I've said, your work should be more than just something to keep you busy from nine to five. Regardless of the degree of commitment you have to your career (and I hope it is very strong), your workplace should reflect your style and taste. Bringing touches from home will make even the most temporary job a bit more meaningful to you. Even a single treasured possession will brighten your office and your attitude.

Certainly when your career is a vital part of your life, and when you find you are putting in more than your required forty hours, your office becomes an important focal point and should provide you with some of the warm feeling you get at home. Having a favorite print on the wall, a special vase on your desk (one you fill with flowers because work is the place you love to be)—these touches make you feel good and tell everyone who enters your turf that you are a thoughtful, concerned person. Keeping makeup and perhaps a change of clothes handy becomes a necessity to maintain your style after hours, when you have no time to go home and change. Being prepared creates confidence; and that confidence takes you through life with great style.

1. Make style a way of life,
not just the clothes you wear.

2. Translate your fashion sense to
your home and your office. Make both places
yours by decorating them in a style
that suits you, and makes you feel good.

3. Entertaining calls for a sense of
style, too, in the way you set a table,
serve a meal, and welcome friends, making
them feel special and at home.

Putting Style to Work for You

ashion makes the strongest style statement and, because your fashion consciousness can be developed without the help of a specialist, fashion awareness is this week's project. Hard as it may be to face, your closet is the place to start.

Maybe it is because we were constantly being told, as children, to clean up our closets that, as adults, we are somewhat less than fastidious where this task is concerned. For some, cleaning out the back part of the closet is much like going on a treasure hunt: things have been back there for so long they look like surprises when they are finally fished out (this is certainly where I go to look for emergency dollar bills and loose change—well, at least those few extra pennies needed to complete a roll of fifty). For others, venturing into the recesses of the closet is more reminiscent of the *Twilight Zone*. Regardless of which category of warrior you fall into, fall into that closet!

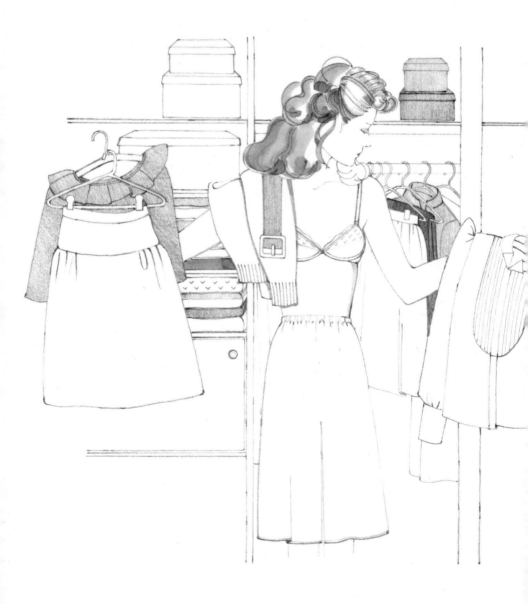

Evacuate the Closet:
a Search and Destroy Mission

The only way to clean a closet properly is to take out every last item, spreading your wardrobe out over bed, chair, and any other available display prop. (Naturally, this is not the thing to do when you have a mere thirty minutes to kill: dedicate the whole day to this one.) The other requisite instruction is what to wear: your best undergarments. Since you will be trying on everything, you should start out prepared, in your best-fitting bra and hose, with a slip close by. You simply cannot truly tell how well a garment looks without the right underpinnings.

Separate your clothes by season: winter, summer, transitional (clothes that take you through spring and fall)

Take a pad and pen and list the garments by season and by classification: skirts/pants/dresses/jackets/blouses/sweaters. One by one, try on each piece. If an item is damaged (ripped or stained, for instance) beyond repair, or if it does not fit, or if it is so outmoded that you can't imagine wearing it again, put it in a discard pile and cross it off the list. If it fits, feels good, and looks fresh (or will with routine cleaning), put on other items to make a complete outfit.

Make lists

Mark each of three pages with one of the seasonal headings. List each complete outfit on the appropriate page. On three other pages, list lone pieces and the garments needed to make complete outfits. Example: Your summer black cotton skirt needs a bold colored top such as a red camisole. When you are finished, you should have six clean lists of completed outfits and sole pieces for each of the three seasons.

SAMPLE "SUMMER" LISTS

Master List in Progress

Completed outfits with accessories:

1) Three-piece cotton knit suit, multicolored print; gray shoes and purse

2) Striped seersucker shirt dress; multicolored sash; white flats; straw bag

3) Navy camisole and skirt; navy sandals and slim-strapped shoulder bag**

4) White trousers and black tank top; cream pumps; black clutch

5) Black cotton skirt and red cotton sweater; black sandals; red purse

6) Plum silk dress; tan pumps and purse

7) Black trousers and pink shirt; black sandals and clutch

** needed

Shopping List in Progress

Lone separates:	Shop for:
1) white cotton skirt	white blouse
	white camisole
2) gray sweater	light gray trousers
3) red miniskirt	red tank top
	plus: navy sandals and shoulder bag

Future purchases:

- another cotton shirt; dress

- a sundress for weekend parties

- a linen suit for special business interviews

Note: as you make purchases, cross items off the "shop" list and add to "complete" list. *Example:* when you buy the white camisole, add "8) white skirt and camisole; white flats; straw bag" to the master list in progress.

Accessorize

Arrange the completed outfits over your furniture (to simulate mannequins) and polish them with accessories. Mark down the shoes, purse, belt and/or scarf needed for each: again put what you have on the outfit lists, what you need on the piece lists.

Keep calm

Don't get hysterical as you return the few complete outfits to the closet. There will be a lot of space on the rods, but this is another case of quality versus quantity. Besides, careful shopping trips will flesh out your wardrobe soon enough.

Shop

The first new clothes to buy are the items needed to make those odd pieces work for you. As you buy them, transfer garments from the "lone separates" list to the "completed outfits" list.

The three complete outfit lists (one for each season) are your master lists. When all the odd separates are acquired, take an overall view of your wardrobe and then decide what else is needed—more dresses or casualwear or whatever.

To avoid winding up with a future discard pile as big as the one you just "destroyed," pay careful attention to future shopping. Buy only complete outfits. If you find yourself saying things like, "Gee, I love this fuschia and ochre skirt—I just know I'll find dozens of tops for it," STOP. If the right blouse or sweater isn't right there, forget it. For all those wondering if you should buy a fuschia and ochre skirt at all (since there is probably only one top that will look right with it, if that) the answer is: if it makes you look good and you really adore it, go ahead. I know that many fashion consultants suggest buying only those clothes that have a high mix-and-match quotient, but few women are truly content with the sameness that the various combinations have. Mix-and-match clothes tend to be neutrals and if you wear neutrals too often, you tend to develop a very neutral (b-l-a-n-d!) image. Just because you're buying separates (a skirt and sweater as opposed to a dress) doesn't mean each piece has to go with other garments—if it works out that way, fine, but don't let that aspiration dictate every purchase you make.

Clothes that work to give you a savvier image, which in turn gives you a boost of self-confidence: that is the goal to set. It does take determination, a lot of it just to keep yourself from putting all those duds back in the closet. Forget the "maybe I'll wear this orange polka dot halter someday" dream and start putting clothes to work for you right now.

Attitude

I n week one, allure meant beauty; in week two, it stood for style. This week, it translates to attitude; the way you project the inner you through your actions and create a mystique or image that piques the interest of others. Attitude means being responsive: how to react as well as act, to keep others interested.

Attitude: Taking Beauty and Style to the Next Dimension

Critics often describe a poor performance by an actor or an actress as two-dimensional—he or she looked correct, but didn't have the liveliness to bring the flat image to life. Unfortunately, many people act out real two-dimensional lives every day. Consider the beautiful woman who lacks the warmth, the humor or the intelligence to merit more than a few lengthy stares: she acts on the belief that her beauty is enough to offer the world. The truth is, others want more than that, and she, in fact, should demand it of herself.

The woman to whom sustained interest is shown will be the one who has an excitement about her, whose zest for life animates her whole being and who shares this electricity with those who touch her. Of course, no one can be "on" twenty-four hours a day; and having to talk yourself into feeling this *joie de vivre* won't make it either—you must truly feel it. But you can genuinely improve your outlook on life much of the time and be the flame that attracts others.

The word that sums up this feeling is attitude.

WORDS TO LIVE BY	WORDS TO FORGET IMMEDIATELY
expressive	shy
able	incompetent
vibrant	timid
alive	passive
go-getter	meek
confident	doubting
positive	critical
assertive	nervous
assured	afraid

How do you get from the right side of the page to the left? COURAGE. You look your fears in the face and dismiss them. That means ignoring nervous cramps, sweaty palms, and a heart beating in double time. The only way to get from A to B is to breathe in, forge ahead, and never turn around. Forcing yourself to accomplish something, to take that first step into unchartered waters gives you a positive self-history to refer to when the time comes for a harder trial. Trust in yourself little by little. There is no other way to overcome fear.

A tangible example.

Suppose that you wanted to become a photographer. You would break down this goal into stages. First, you would trade in your instamatic for a better camera—not the top of the line, but one you could manage—and learn how it works. Second, you would shoot a few rolls of film (black and white because it holds many advantages for the newcomer), examine your shots, experiment with different film speeds and lenses. Third, you would look for more serious subjects to please a critical eye. Then you would look for a first assignment: volunteer to take the pictures at a wedding or graduation. If you are good, these samples of your work will lead to a paying job, such as taking a formal portrait or shooting another party. Each step is an accomplishment that leads you to the next stage, giving you confidence and credentials.

Use this same logical progression to accomplish the more personal goals of self-improvement. If you aren't happy with your personality, with your job, or with your pizzazz quotient, ask yourself why. Make a list, then tackle it. Don't give in to discontent by succumbing to feelings of inferiority, depression, confusion, frustration. If you feel that you're not smart enough to be outgoing, select a subject of genuine interest to you and bone up on it (see the next chapter for ideas). If you feel depressed, pinpoint the cause (lack of success at the office; losing an important relationship) and set goals to get yourself moving on the right track (learn a job-related skill; take steps to improve your social life). Taking positive action—DOING—when facing a negative situation always improves your outlook and attitude. Negative inaction—being depressed—never does.

Very often, a woman keeps herself from projecting an outgoing personality from plain and simple fear rather than a rational reason. You stop yourself from joining a lively group at a party not because you aren't intelligent enough, but because you *fear* you aren't intelligent enough. You are afraid of the possibility that you won't be accepted, even though you have no concrete reason for the feeling. And just what would happen if you were given the cold shoulder? You'd simply find another group to join! Unfortunately, rational thinking fades as your wild imagination runs rampant: you picture fellow partygoers hurling insults or their drinks at you. But, objectively, what are the chances of this happening? Nonexistent. (No matter how mismannered some people have become, no one is that boorish, at least not after the third grade.) In fact, most partygoers have a the-more-the-merrier philosophy that welcomes all others into their circle. All you have to do is try.

You want to get over irrational fears and develop the assertive attitude that gets you to make the first move, to reach out to others, to display your sense of humor or warmth or intellect. Because if you wait for the world to notice you, you're going to be very lonely. You have to reach out and tap the world on its shoulder to announce your presence. If not, all you will have are regrets.

SUMMARY OF DAY FIFTEEN

1. Start to face your fears by rationally breaking them down and analyzing the components.
You'll see that you don't have any good reason to be afraid, to not try for accomplishments.

2. Don't let the past keep you from moving forward. All that exists for you to achieve should tempt you to attempt.

3. Attempt, regardless of the possibility of failure, and you won't fail.

4. Trust in yourself and believe in your self-worth. Sit down and make a list of your virtues. Read it aloud whenever you feel insecure.

DAY 16

Be Interesting

The easiest way to feel confident about yourself is to know that you have something to feel proud of and to offer to others. A sense of humor, an amusing wit, a giving heart are even more important than a medical or legal degree. Sharing your special qualities makes you interesting to others, distinguishes you.

Making Yourself Interesting

In addition to personal qualities, being interesting means being knowledgeable in a unique way and knowing how to captivate an audience. Reciting the capitals of all fifty states indicates knowledge, but is not as interesting as describing the capitals of all the South Pacific islands. Being different from the rest is what makes you stand out in a crowded room or on a busy street. Of course, the difference must be charismatic to provoke interest, not just curious stares. Here are four ways to make that difference.

1. Reading

How often do you take the time to read a newspaper, front page to last? No, you don't have to be a walking, talking wire service, but keeping up on current affairs is a must, something too few women make time for. For your own satisfaction, you should know about the world around you. Every morning, spend a few minutes, at the very least, reading the headlines and first two paragraphs of the prominent articles. On Sunday, try to buy one of the country's top papers (*The New York Times, The Washington Post, Los Angeles Times*) and read through the business, book review, and week in review sections.

Read the classics, one every two weeks. Being an English Lit major in college, I grew to loathe the very word *classics*. But now that I can read an eighteenth- or nineteenth-century novel and know that there is no assignment attached to it, the reading is pure pleasure.

Investigate a nonfiction topic that interests you by reading a book on it. One of the bestsellers on investing will prove to be a challenge, not a bore—and every woman should know that "investments" mean more than a passbook savings account. (Did you know that you could invest in a penny stock and triple your money if it goes from one cent to three? Something to consider for the beginning investor.)

2. Travel

If you like traveling, start being more adventuresome. Use an inexpensive package deal to get you to a new place, then use your ingenuity to seek out different attractions. Skip the usual half-day tour of the city and rent a car or car-and-driver to show you the more unusual places—your hotel manager can tell you which local neighborhoods are truly reflective of the country or region you're in; explain that you want to see true "local color," not the diluted tourist version. Visit the nearest university and talk with students. Converse with a hopeful artist at a museum. While away an hour at a rustic pub or sidewalk café and "absorb" the atmosphere.

Take advantage of a vacation to shed the inhibitions that keep the woman you long to be hidden back home. Be daring in a new way, knowing that, as a stranger, you are starting from scratch as you make new acquaintances. With no one to judge you, you are free to project whatever image you like. You will be surprised at how natural your secret persona feels and will hopefully take this "new woman" home with you.

Note: foreign travel is very exotic and does require you to be a latter-day explorer, open-minded and curious; if this sounds too grand for you right now, remember that you needn't leave the U.S. to enjoy a sense of adventure—travel to the nearest big city or to the next state, if you like. Any new surroundings provide fertile ground for trying on your new image.

If you aren't wild about traveling, or can't yet afford the trip you'd love to take, become an armchair traveler. Travel books and slides which can often be rented or borrowed from a foreign country's board of tourism *are* the next best thing to being there. And this "research" will help you decide where you would most like to travel in the future.

3. Developing your creativity

No one is without a creative talent. So you never took to the piano as a child—that doesn't mean you are hopeless. There is something about practicing under a mother's or teacher's watchful eye that creates a loathing of the otherwise harmless playing of the scales. Consider taking up the piano, or any other instrument (my secret dream is to play the harp—how beautiful!), and set your own practice schedule—Mother will be surprised by how well you stick to it.

If you feel music is for listening, not making, consider the arts—not trekking through museums, but trying your own hand. Oil or watercolor painting, sculpture, printmaking, stained glass, origami, collage, drawing, cartooning—these are only some of the choices that allow your imagination to run in a positive direction. Writing, whether you tackle a book, a song, or a commercial jingle, is another gratifying form of expression. So are dance (ballet, tap, jazz), and the theater arts.

Concentrate on having fun and exploring your range of talents. Don't worry about being "good enough." You are the only audience you must please in this endeavor. Self-expression is something you do for you. If you aren't satisfied with your results at first, you will be with dedication and perseverance. Whether you keep your creativity to yourself or decide to share it with others, developing it is a must for encouraging feelings of self-esteem and for making "yes, I can do it" your answer when facing a new challenge.

4. Be spontaneous; be daring

Explore the unexplored—you needn't travel to the Serengeti; a local playhouse or cabaret will do for starters.

Are you basically dull? Answer these questions. If you and a friend are to meet for dinner, is it always the friend who must suggest the place? If you are trapped indoors because of rain that has spoiled picnic plans, how quickly would you devise an alternate activity? Can you pack a suitcase on a moment's notice or do you agonize for weeks?

If you are unable to take fast, positive action in each of these instances, you are in a rut, and that is not interesting!

Dull people wear the same hairstyle month in and year out; they rarely try a new shade of lipstick just for the fun of it; they tell the same anecdotes over and over. If this sounds too familiar, you need a shake-up. Allure means having that vital spark, that energy and enthusiasm to be daring.

It might seem to be a contradiction in terms, but spontaneity does call for advance planning; it is a habit you develop. Investigate goings-on in your city: you must know what the options are before you can pick one. Read new restaurant, club and cabaret/theater reviews. Keep a file that tells you when the skating rink is open, when a rock group or jazz trio is coming to town. Make sure that your wardrobe is well maintained so that you can change clothes quickly if the picnic becomes a grown-ups' trip to the circus.

If you have that spark, that difference that makes you the one others turn to for excitement, you'll be truly interesting.

Challenging Yourself

Being satisfied with yourself is perhaps the most deadly fate of all. Don't misunderstand: you should always feel good about yourself, but not complacent, and never so smug that you think there's nothing left to learn. There is always something new to do or to read or to try. Be the first to go wind tunnel flying or rent a hot air balloon for an afternoon. Learn to rewire a lamp or build a bookcase. Produce your own cable show on a free public access station or start a newsletter on a subject you want to know more about.

Above all, never let yourself become idle because that is the foundation of dullness. And that's not what you want for yourself.

The Makings of Good Conversation

There are two basic types of conversation: superficial talk and serious discussion. You should be able to master both.

Superficial talk starts new friendships, makes anxious moments easier (example: waiting in a doctor's office), acts as a warm-up to more enjoyable discussion. It is hard to ask probing questions of a casual acquaintance: you must use the superficial to help a conversation progress.

Superficial conversation is everyday conversation: "Hi, how are you?" and "How was your day?" Yet it needn't be insipid. To overcome the superficiality of these questions, you must ask them with genuine interest and answer the same way, with more than a casual "Fine" or "The usual." Tell an amusing story or confide an unusual incident. Wait for a comment and take the conversation one step further. To move from superficial to serious, those engaged in discussion must take turns strengthening the content of the talk. If not, you never make it past the banalities.

Small talk is hard to carry off well because it easily becomes boring. People who dislike cocktail parties, for instance, are really saying that they dislike small talk, the cocktail party mainstay. But if you are interested in forming new friendships and widening your circle of acquaintances, you need to master "beginner conversations." Acceptable topics for superficial talk include current music, books, fashion, art trends, travel, money, television ("Do you own a Beta or VHS?") and food—everything from the latest gourmet market to the best place for take-out Chinese. (Some things never change.)

The key to developing superficial conversations is asking questions. Get the other person talking, fuel the conversation with questions and then offer opinions: take the initiative and let the other person run with it (people adore talking about themselves, their preferences). Look for openings to inch the conversation closer to a topic that interests you. This provides a mutually satisfying exchange, the perfect foundation for serious conversation.

Serious conversation is something you slip into, like an icy swimming pool. Because it calls for revealing personal opinions and emotions, you can't jump right in. At the start of a conversation, your protective force field is activated. As the superficial talk progresses, you make decisions about sharing your innermost thoughts and the shield falls away, enabling you to touch on more meaningful ideas.

Trust in yourself not only to form opinions, but to express them. At work, this means suggesting ideas, not just nodding in agreement. At play, this means exchanging points of view and debating them. Develop in yourself the strength of conviction to stick to your beliefs and the ability to articulate them to make yourself a woman of substance.

SUMMARY OF DAY SIXTEEN

1. Make yourself interesting by exploring new avenues of interest.

2. Rediscover reading, an excellent way to develop your thought processes.

3. Always challenge yourself to try more things.

4. Conversation is an art: improve your "small talk" ability and express more important thoughts when you have an opportunity to deepen a conversation.

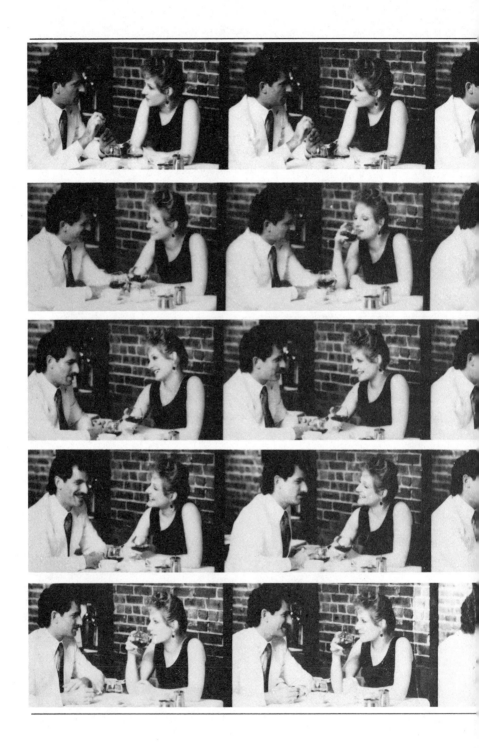

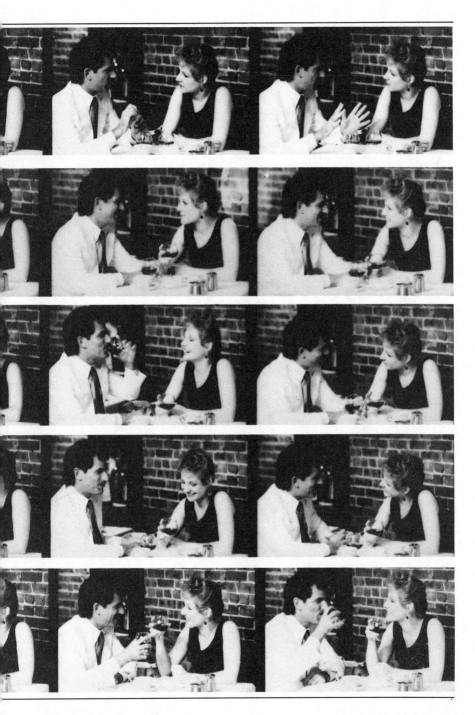

Chemistry in action.

Be Interested

Knowing how to listen is as vital to a conversation as knowing what to say. It is unfair to ask a question only to close your ears and tune out the answer, as for instance many do when they ask "How are you?" Interest is give-and-take: you create it by listening and responding. Giving someone your attention is a much appreciated gift, a quality that speaks well of you.

There's no doubt that we are all hard pressed for time in today's world. We each have lists of things that must be done, yet we never get to them—letters needing replies collect dust, stacks of messages pile up, calls wait to be returned. Operating fifteen miles above the speed limit, today's woman doesn't have the time to stop, assess, relax, and listen. Too many friendships are carried on via ten minute phone calls; love relationships, if not serious, fall by the wayside or, if there is a chemistry, must bloom overnight—there's no time for courtship. Consequently, you never get past the superficial because you don't take the time to listen and respond.

For many, a readjustment of priorities is in order. Put people at the top of your list; without friends and lovers, when you do come up for air, you'll have the sense that life is whirring by you, not that you are in the center of it.

How to Listen

Listening is accomplished by being aware. Develop a natural curiosity that gets you to ask questions and investigate. Your questions give others the opportunity to express themselves and put you in a flattering light.

Listening is accomplished by paying attention and retaining information. Do you recall a personal opinion a good friend expressed to you in your last conversation? Do you remember her favorite color? A lover's secret passion? Your co-workers' birthdays? These details might seem trivial, but knowing the "little things" about a friend makes the friend feel special. Don't you feel terrific when a special someone remembers your perfume or favorite flower?

When interacting with others, offer your full concentration. When talking on the telephone, be sure that one ear isn't listening to the TV or that you aren't trying to simultaneously read a book.

Listening is accomplished through body language. When conversing in person, maintain that all-important eye contact. Be certain that your eyes aren't more absorbed in your surroundings than in the expressions and gestures of your companion(s).

Other elements of body language convey interest, too. Keep your hands visible: hiding them under the dinner table, for example, is distracting. Turn your body toward the other person to create the impression of forming your own sphere. Maintain an "open" stance: avoid crossing arms and legs in a tight, defensive position.

Listening is accomplished by understanding. Before you respond to what has been said, think about the statement and take the time to formulate your response. Make sure you comprehend the dialogue and that your answer will relate to it, especially if you are one of the many victims of foot-in-mouth disease (symptom: you often, and disastrously, say the first thing that pops into your head). Witty repartee is terrific, but it is a skill that de-velops with maturity; unless you were born with a silver tongue, think first, speak second. You won't be penalized for not being fast on the draw, but rather complimented for being thoughtful and concerned.

Most importantly, listening is accomplished by response. Exam-ple: a friend tells you about a difficult situation at her office. The interested response offers a suggestion or solution; the disin-terested response switches the conversation to a problem of your own.

Your response must directly relate to what has been said. The "I can top that" answer keeps a conversation from being mutually satisfying. A good listener can tell when no words are needed, when a look that says "I understand" or a hug is the desired reaction. Many situations defy easy answers; pat solu-tions ("It'll be okay" and "time will tell" are two examples of the highest form of superficiality) are the worst. Personal experience is helpful if your anecdote draws a parallel to the issue at hand.

A good dialogue involves a steady progression from one topic to another. But an abrupt change in subject is not an ap-propriate response. Example: if a man tells you of his love of golf and you respond by confessing ignorance and asking him to ex-plain the game to you, you've demonstrated interest. But if you tell him you prefer water-skiing and launch into your recent trip to Florida, you've not only shown a lack of interest, but a lack of good manners as well. No, you needn't listen to endless talk of eagles and birdies, but if you want to tactfully switch the subject, you need to find a bridge. Example: "I'd like to try golf at least once, but my current passion is for water sports. Have you ever tried skiing?" The bridge enables you to guide the conversation so that it is mutually satisfying and provides a steady exchange of information and thought, keeping a conversation interesting for both of you.

Once you learn how to listen, you will know better how to respond: with humor, with sympathy, with an opinion, an anec-dote, or with only a smile, an expression that never fails to say, "I'm interested."

SUMMARY OF DAY SEVENTEEN

1. Show interest by developing your
curiosity and asking questions.

2. Learn to listen: don't fall victim
to the in-one-ear-out-the-other way of life.

3. Listening is accomplished by being aware,
paying attention, projecting correct body
language, understanding and careful response.

DAY 18

How to Project at Work

Personal drive, that inner motivation that pushes you to attempt the unknown, determines whether you have great ambition or the more easily attainable contentment with work. Ambition is not the dirty word some people would have you believe; it is not without the feeling of satisfaction, but is a satisfaction that keeps pushing you ahead to greater highs. On the other hand, there is nothing lacking in the woman who is not working her way up the ladder, the woman who is happy with her position; to maintain her satisfaction, she will still need to push herself toward new challenges, or else lose much of her contentment and feel herself sinking into a rut. Whether you strive to increase your wpm at the typewriter (or, more likely, the keyboard!), to write and deliver better speeches, or to boost your high-level profit margin, keep your work exciting. This increases your motivation to go to work every day, creates a company-wide enthusiasm for your input, and gives you the praise we all so need to hear (and, in more capitalist terms, praise leads to raise).

Take Charge Attitude: Turning a Job into a Career

Regardless of how ambitious you are, the work you do should have all the qualities of a career, not merely a job (translated: drudge). Just look at the definitions. A job is a "small miscellaneous piece of work." A career is the "pursuit of consecutive progressive achievement." Which would you rather wake at seven a.m. for?

Every occupation can be rewarding and fun. Don't let the "I'm just" syndrome keep you from these goals. Example: resist saying "I'm just a receptionist. Why should I do more than answer the phone?" Instead say "I can make my work as a receptionist more challenging by taking on a new responsibility." Or, if you don't want to stop at being a receptionist, look around your company for options that will take you beyond the front desk. If, for example, you work at a law firm, find out about working in the law library, about doing research, about taking an evening course in paralegal training or in pre-law, if your aspirations go higher.

If you keep challenging yourself, your days will be so filled that five o'clock surprises you every afternoon. But if you spend the better part of your day just passing time, it will seem as though that clock hand never moves.

Presenting Your Ideas

To feel part of a firm or company, you should get involved, and know its inner workings. Depending on your position you might often be called on for your input. Taking the initiative is, however, another option to consider and can help your career. Opportunity doesn't always knock—sometimes you must invite it over.

To present your ideas, you really have to be a salesperson.

You need to finely hone your presentation. First, clearly organize your thoughts on paper or on a cassette (the latter, played back, lets you hear how you sound and make any necessary adjustments for the presentation). Second, play an adult version of "let's pretend." In your mind's eye, or by talking it out, pretend that you are speaking and anticipate a wide variety of reactions—play devil's advocate with yourself. If you are well prepared, you will have a smart (not smart aleck) response for any point that might be raised.

Be prepared to implement your ideas, too. If you suggest switching from the postal service to an overnight express outfit, be ready to supply names of potential companies and to get the system into operation.

Projecting Yourself in a Meeting

Having to speak in front of a group is at the top of nearly everyone's fear list. Recognize that you always face disagreement in your personal and professional life, but this is merely an exchange of thought to arrive at the best possible conclusion. No one will throw rotten tomatoes at you! In fact, she who has the courage and enterprise to stand up is more often envied than shot down.

Getting over the Jitters

Whether you voice a question at a meeting or are the principal speaker, be prepared with written notes. A few professional speakers can wing it; most of us can't. If you have notes to refer to, whether or not you actually use them, you will be less anxious.

Know Your Audience

Get into the habit of greeting your co-workers by their full names, rather than with a vague "Good morning" (which on its own usually comes out half mumbled). Recognizing faces when

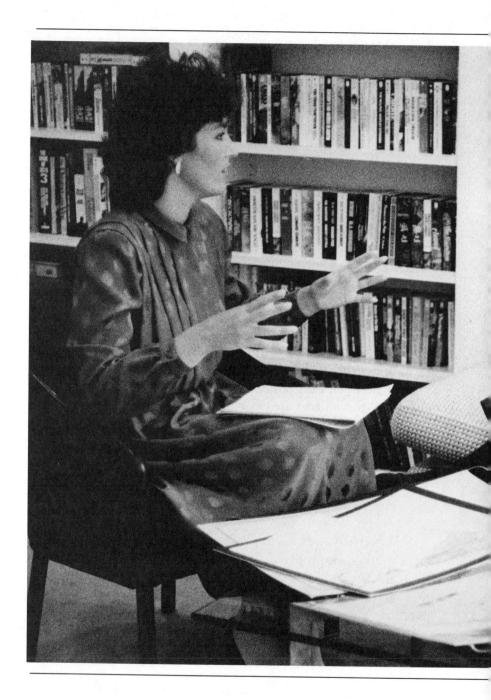

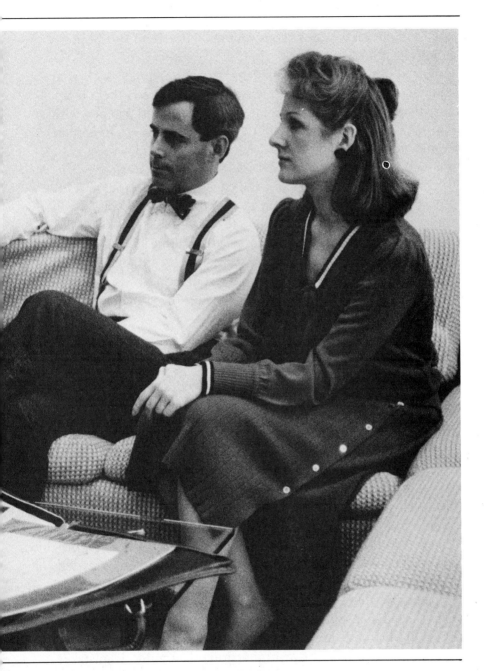

Elaine holds her audience's attention with
her enthusiasm and a clear, concise outline of
her ideas. (Note her excellent posture!)

you look out on a crowd keeps your audience from resembling a hungry group of cannibals.

If you are giving a lecture to strangers, mingle with your audience beforehand to get a sense of what interests them most.

If you are sitting in on a meeting, bring a pad and pen with you. Make notes for yourself. Write down the most important points others make. That way when you have an idea to express, you will be sure to respond exactly to the issue.

Being prepared gives you the edge over fear or nervous jitters. However, sometimes they do get the better of you. If you can't conquer them, learn to hide them. A smile will keep your lips from quivering. Sitting will steady shaking knees (though standing is more authoritative, a strong voice can help make up the difference). And, after making your remarks, asking for questions from the group or audience takes the pressure off you.

Getting Ahead

The real world is not as logical as most of us would like. We think that if we work hard we will progress in a steady manner. That doesn't always happen. And when it doesn't, frustration and resentment builds. If you haven't been getting the promotions you want, don't lose heart and berate yourself. Take action instead.

Ask your boss or supervisor for the requirements to get to the level you want. Ask for constructive criticism—what you haven't been doing that you should or what you could be doing better. And listen. Don't rush to your defense with excuses. Listen, understand and then comment: outline your plan of revised action and ask for encouragement. Remember that your boss is not (usually) there to keep you down: his/her employees' performance is a direct reflection of him/her. You won't be chewed out for asking how to improve your work.

Projecting the right mental attitude is a must. If mistakes are pointed out to you, resist putting yourself down. An imperfect job performance is not a reflection of your worth. It is a catalyst to get you to try harder. Think of your positive accomplishments and realize that making mistakes is the only way to get ahead.

Maintaining your self-esteem is vital. Don't lose sight of it—that's what got you to ask what you were doing wrong and what will get you to work harder to get the "job" done right, to get ahead to where you want to be.

```
┌─────────────SUMMARY OF DAY EIGHTEEN─────────────┐
│                                                  │
│   1. To challenge yourself, turn your job into   │
│   a career. Look for lateral growth if climbing the │
│   corporate ladder is not in your game plan.     │
│                                                  │
│   2. Become a doer, not a follower, at the       │
│   office. This boosts your position, but even    │
│   more important, your self-confidence quotient. │
│                                                  │
│   3. Take action to get ahead. Don't wait for    │
│   someone to discover you: make your presence known. │
│                                                  │
└──────────────────────────────────────────────────┘
```

How to Project at Play

You can make excitement happen. Whether you initiate a conversation with a new acquaintance at a party, take the swimming lessons you've been promising yourself for years, or dazzle guests at a covered dish supper with a majestic chocolate soufflé, you have the potential to be the woman who attracts attention by projecting an outgoing attitude.

Making Playtime Count

If you are as dedicated to your career as most women are (and should be), leisure time is short, and you have to make the most of it. First, get organized. One woman I know procrastinates so about straightening up her apartment that she puts aside every Saturday afternoon, passing up all invitations on the excuse of doing her chores. The worst part is that come Saturday, she fritters away the day, without any of the cleaning getting done. She needs to readjust her schedule: laundry one evening, shopping for food on the way home the next night and picking up after herself a little each day.

Second, improve the quality of your weekends and evenings. Make the reservations for that ski weekend and find out once and for all what schussing means. Reacquaint yourself with your jogging shoes. Call a friend and explore a new antiquing town in the country. If you're single, improving your social life will bring you into contact with new men. If you're married or involved, your newfound zest will renew the initial excitement you felt when you and he first met and discovered each other.

Third, take chances. Start doing things you've dreamed about, yet never dared to do. You aren't too old or too fat or too tall or too tired or too whatever excuse you've been using to stay sedate and sedentary. Zap yourself into action. And so what if you fall flat on your face—chances are this won't happen, yet if it did, it would be far superior to never having tried at all. Yes, you will tumble into bed, exhausted at the end of the day—and have the best night's sleep ever.

Developing the Attitude

There are three key attitudes that guarantee attention and success in social situations. The one you choose depends on how confident you are.

High drama seems audacious at first glance, but is actually an approach for the very shy. By acting a bit outrageous, you draw attention to yourself: others take notice of you without your having to approach them directly.

At a party, you would bring your host an eye-catching gift—anything from a single calla lily to a double-magnum of wine (depending on your budget). At a restaurant, you would order a dramatic dish, one that is prepared at your table (thereby creating a great commotion) or a sumptuous chocolate dessert bound to create interest. At the beach, you would build a sand-castle—and have everyone offering to help.

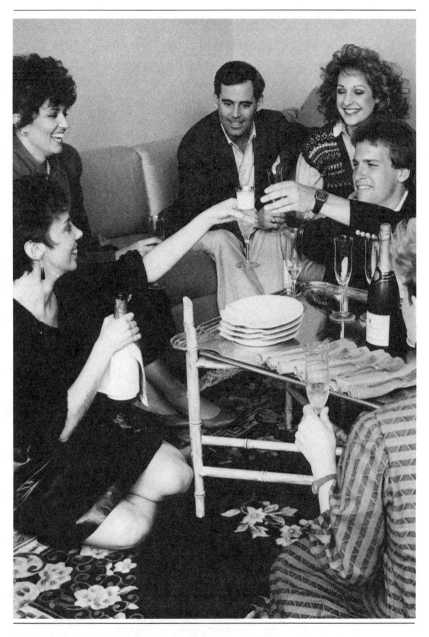

Champagne is the perfect attention-getter.
And it needn't be expensive: look for sparkling wine
bottled by the *methode champenoise*—champagne
grapes grown outside the champagne region of France,
but often just as delicious when served icy cold.

People are attracted by the energy a high drama person radiates; it is a powerful magnet used by the famous and the celebrated, equally available to you. Just be sure that your body language is inviting, not intimidating as self-confidence often is, especially to women. Smile warmly, look interested and right into the eyes of others, not past them.

The gregarious nature initiates contact with easy openers such as "How do you know our hostess?" or "Isn't this a great apartment?" at a party, and "That dish looks delicious—may I ask what it is?" to the man at the next table in a restaurant. At the beach, you would ask for volunteers to start that sandcastle.

The outgoing woman doesn't want to wait for others to get up the courage to talk to her; she goes after them. People are attracted by the self-assurance they wish they had and are flattered that you sought them out, grateful not to have to make the first move themselves. If you are great at small talk or can tell an amusing anecdote, this approach is effective.

The organizer is deceptively bold. She uses props for attention, appearing at first to hide behind them. In reality, it takes great daring to put her skills into play. At a party, this woman artfully arranges a platter of hors d'oeuvres for the host and initiates conversations as she offers it to other guests. One friend has singlehandedly brought back party games, devising intricate projects guests sometimes prepare for in advance—her ingenuity is the talk of every gathering! At a restaurant, she will offer suggestions to other diners as they peruse the menu and at the beach, she will carve the path to the ocean for your sandcastle. The trick here is to temper your assistance: once you've circulated that platter of mushrooms and dip, and met everyone, turn the reins of the party back to the hostess and pick up a promising conversation.

How to Approach a Man

Few women take the initiative to start a conversation with a man they find interesting—they are as shy about this in the secure setting of a friend's house as they are alone on a tropical island. They let their fear of rejection and their shyness stand in the way. They don't realize that, after a decade or two of dating, many men are even more fearful of rejection and even more shy than they are. Consequently, an opportunity to meet a new man fizzles out.

One of the reasons men say they don't make the first move as often as they'd like is because women make themselves unapproachable. *Example:* Many women dream of that chance meeting that will produce Mr. Right. But most chance meetings occur in the least likely places—the laundromat, the car wash, the token booth in the subway. And in most of these situations, a man who says even the simplest hello is often suspect. *Solution:* There is no doubt that crime has put women at a grave disadvantage, yet not every stranger is a potential criminal. Don't let down all your defenses, but practice being more objective: give the man with initiative a chance.

Of course, both the new male shyness and the female defensiveness lead to one conclusion: start taking the initiative yourself. You have, by now, the self-assurance and the self-confidence to know how great you are: start telling the rest of the world.

Taking the initiative can be as subtle as using body language to show interest: let your eyes speak their magic language for you; be sure your smile is inviting and that you are standing or sitting proudly. This is often all the "invitation" a perceptive man needs.

Starting a conversation is the next step, and is far easier than most people think. Don't worry about being incredibly witty or bright: act naturally and seize a handy subject. Example: at the supermarket, point out the better brand of paper towel to an interesting eligible; at a bookstore, compare writers in the mystery section; in traffic, roll down your window and comment on the music the man in the car next to you is listening to. Be daring enough to strike up a dialogue: men love it. A woman who is adventurous, confident and quite simply "fun," is attractive to the opposite sex.

On those first dates, make sure you listen when he speaks and comment carefully: this avoids those awful lapses in conversation that occur when people give pat, one-word answers. Distinguish yourself by doing the unusual: don't wait for him to send flowers—if you really had a great time, say it with a beautifully written and scented note or a basket of brownies left on his doorstep. Always remember that you can make things happen for yourself; no one else has the vested interest in your life that you do. Make the most of it.

How to Make Friends of Women

No matter how fleeting the moment is, there comes a time when every woman fantasizes about being the only female on earth. Though we try to band together as a "sisterhood" fighting for our equality, we each face competition with other women every day, be it for professional position, for a man's attention, for wealth, for status, even for that last pair of beige pumps at the shoe sale.

One of the great rewards of experiencing self-esteem is that other women do become less threatening: you know your personal worth and hope others can feel the same way about themselves. Yet the self-confident woman runs the risk of appearing smug, and a threat to other women, envious or insecure.

With care, your allure can serve as an example, rather than intimidation. Start by making yourself more approachable. Look into the other woman's eyes as you greet her or talk with her. Offer the same interest you show to a man. Be secure in yourself so that hearing about her accomplishments does not lead you to an interior dialogue of self-doubt. You needn't make another woman feel better by putting yourself down (as some women do), but show signs that you are just as human as she is: lipstick that needs reapplying; a hint (for your sake, only a hint!) of jitters about the situation that has brought you together; revealing a personal opinion that helps you get past the superficial talk.

The reason to bother is basic: closeness with a good woman friend is a wonderful relationship to have. A woman's sensitivity is in perfect balance with a man's pragmatism: both sides are vital and different—women may not always offer more comfort than men, but it is definitely a different kind of comfort.

Yes, there are some women who insist they relate best with men. But more often than not, the reason for this is a negative reflection of the inner self: these women are too insecure about their own merit and, viewing other women as threatening, avoid them. Their relationships with men serve more to bolster their waning egos than as true friendships. Being able to develop strong friendships with women is not only mutually gratifying, but also a sign of your own self-esteem. This companionship will also encourage you to make the most of your social life without having to wait for a man to call.

SUMMARY OF DAY NINETEEN

1. Make excitement happen: take steps to actively plan your social life. Be daring: do things on your own, just for the fun of it.

2. Develop your social persona. Bring the same enthusiasm you bring to your career to your private time. Be more gregarious, more outgoing, more outrageous to distinguish yourself.

3. Take the initiative when the opportunity to meet a new man presents itself. Stop letting fear of rejection keep you from reaching out and showing interest: genuine feelings need to be shared.

4. Court the friendship of women: don't let your new self-confidence set up barriers against this important aspect of your life.

DAY 20

Your Many Faces

The dimensions of allure change as the emphasis of a woman's life changes from career to home to romance. What makes a woman alluring in the bedroom is naturally far different than the look of allure she carries to the office and the one she wears to lunch with a friend. You must distinguish the needs for each occasion as well as move easily from one into the next.

Allure at the office calls for the appropriate clothes for your position. You might not have a change of attire for every day of the week, but you always look correct, "pulled together." This grooming extends to your makeup and your nails: the office is no place to repair chipped polish. Do not wear too much jewelry; keep shoes diligently shined.

You should be as organized with your paperwork as you are with your appearance: a neat briefcase. A brightly colored, oversized portfolio takes the place of those mannish and cumbersome black cases.

Your style is reflected in your professional attitude. You display a winning smile, a straightforward gaze and a firm hand-shake. Consideration when dealing with others is also a high priority. Your enthusiasm should be reflected in your dedication. Personal phone calls are limited to maintain your concentration. Be punctual when you are visited as well as when you have out-side appointments: a great indicator of confidence and ability.

The allure of a lover is, in part, silky lingerie, the lingering scent of perfume, half-closed eyes. But there is more. Touching is the intimate communication that comes before everything else. It is cuddling in the morning—sensual before sexual, always before words, even "good morning." At night, it is dressing up to be undressed: the chignon later unpinned, the camisole later unlaced.

The bedroom is the perfect forum for the unexpected, the outrageous, from champagne chilling to a violinist who knows when to leave. Planning shouldn't be overlooked: the freshest sheets, the smell of fresh flowers, as important if you are married to keep loving special.

Allure means different things to different men. Asking your lover what he finds exciting and irresistible is the best way to be as provocative as you can. As always, listen. Then suggest, dis-cuss.

When women become wives and mothers, they often be-lieve they shouldn't be as sensual as they were before marriage. To keep a marriage vital and interesting as the newness fades, maintaining and projecting the allure of a lover is needed. You are still a woman, not hired household help. Be careful not to trade in your lace teddies for head-to-toe flannel; of course, the old cold-cream-and-curlers image has almost disappeared, but watch out for its replacements: electric rollers and instant face masques still belong in the bathroom.

Keep developing yourself, even if your career is in the home. For most women, it is not enough to be the woman behind the man, no matter how dazzling a prize you are. Independence is alluring: it keeps him on his toes, too.

Homemaker has replaced that full-of-awful-images word "housewife," yet the picture is often the same: housecoat or plaid-shirt-and-khakis uniform that is unflattering for anything other than washing floors. Don't let domestic life rob you of your style, certainly not after six p.m., when your husband comes home. Yes, this is something you do for him, but do it for yourself even more, to keep up your self-image. Only you can turn yourself into a drudge; marriage by itself is not the culprit.

When you are entertaining or socializing with friends, be as sparkling and charismatic as you were when you were single. Just because you have your man doesn't mean you should let yourself become dull—the surest way to lose him. Flirting, for some, is a tantalizing activity; it has a charming quality when kept light (sexual *innuendo, not* advance). Flirting with your husband should be explored, too. Offer your best sexy look across his parents' dining room table; steal a kiss as you wait on line for a movie. It is far easier to be daring with a man you know well: his likes and tastes are familiar; you risk less, try more.

As a marriage progresses, there is less discovery; you no longer hang onto his every word; one evening, you find that you can read a book and converse with him at the same time. These are signs that your allure quotient needs a rise. Start giving him the attention you did when the romance was new; make a date to meet for lunch; meet at his office after your workday, theater tickets in hand. Keeping yourself and your marriage vital prevents it from becoming routine. If it is routine already, shake it up. (This is true of any long-standing relationship.)

Motherhood is not synonymous with lackluster either. Taste and style are developed at a very young age. Smart-looking activewear, especially when coordinated with your child's clothes, keeps you looking savvy and instills a sense of appearance in your child. Don't sacrifice bedroom allure; if it makes you more comfortable, keep it behind closed doors, but keep it in your life.

Maintain your interests after motherhood, to keep yourself interesting to your husband and friends—endless talk of offspring is not forever alluring. Remember that you are more than a wife and a mother: you are a woman first.

One of the first "roles" you played as a child often loses its importance in adult life; this is a mistake. Friendships are a gratifying facet of life, even though career and love become greater concerns. *The allure of a friend* is more founded in personality than your other roles, certainly where initial interest is concerned. A striking appearance is often what first fascinates a man; the appropriate appearance is the first impression an employer makes. Friendships begin at the sight of a smile, not the mouth-watering lip gloss that smile might be decorated with. Because other feelings and responses are activated in friendships, especially those between women, maintaining the "allure" of a friendship rests on other criteria.

A close friend should be compassionate and supportive, without being judgmental. She must know how to listen and to respond with concern and feeling. She is there for the fun times as well as the difficult ones. A friend is not to be taken advantage of: called on when a date cancels, or ignored when romance blooms.

Because friendships do not rely on the energy of a sexual attraction or office accomplishments, as most love affairs and careers respectively do, trust is even more important in this relationship. This is a bond that gives a beginning acquaintance the dimension it needs to take on greater meaning.

Acquaintances—the people you would add to a guest list after your closest must-haves were all included—act on a different dynamism. The relationship is lighter, almost superficial. Being bubbly and bright and presenting a snazzy image makes you a perfect candidate for being an acquaintance, and qualifies best under the heading of a "role" you might play. Being a good guest and, when situations are reversed, a good hostess exhibits your allure.

To take you from one relationship to another, you need to make subtle adjustments. The proper office blouse opens at the neckline before dinner with your husband. The flirting smile and twinkling eyes you show off at a party grow serious with concern as you converse with a friend. The measured handshake replaces the tender caress you gave your lover as the clock strikes nine a.m. and your first appointment arrives at your office. The stylish jogging suit slips over your camisole and tap pants for an outing with your child. Makeup is removed to reveal only fresh skin as you immerse yourself in concentration at the potter's wheel.

Once you develop your sense of allure, you gently alter it to suit the different aspects of your life. You do not have to learn a new allure for each occasion; it is the same innate feeling, but with slight variations in its projection.

SUMMARY OF DAY TWENTY

1. Allure means different signals at different times. Know what is appropriate to each occasion.

2. Learn to make readjustments in your image projection as you live out each day.

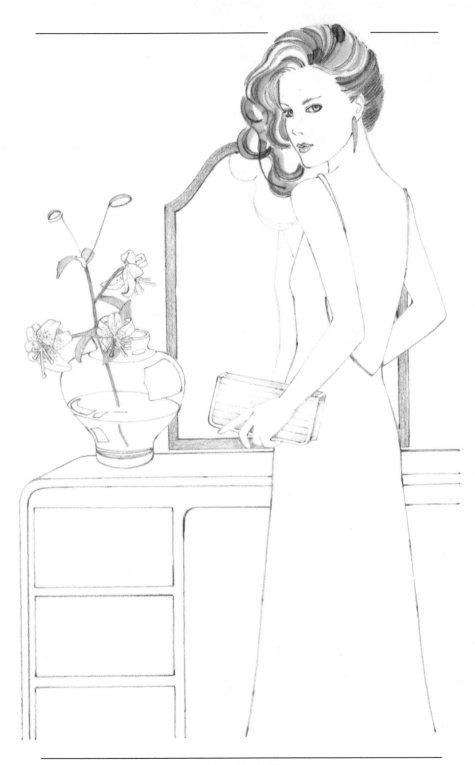

DAY 21

Putting It All Together

Today is not another lesson; it is a day to assess, to evaluate what you have absorbed, to determine what must still be accomplished. Allure is not a list of twenty-one items to remember; it is a quality that should be second nature to you, reflected in everything you do. Allure calls for conscious decision making—every time you open your closet for something to wear; every time you take someone's hand in yours—but the answers become more obvious, more natural as time goes on.

To evaluate your progress, look over the summary of each of the past twenty days. Are the concepts clear to you? If not, read through the chapters to clarify their meaning. Understanding is vital.

Put what you've learned to work. It is no longer enough to say your "I'm terrific's" in the bathroom mirror, it is time to say them through everything you do, to the world. After practicing your best eye expressions, start to use them every day—maintaining direct eye contact during introductions and conversations is the simplest gesture you can make and will have the most impact: everyone responds favorably to receiving undivided attention. Once you feel secure and successful with the basic expressions, you will have the confidence to try the more playful ones.

Set up a timetable for accomplishments. List five things you want to achieve: anything from taking ceramics lessons to getting a raise to meeting new friends to throwing a fabulous party to discovering a new romance. Give each a priority number and then list the steps that will put each into reach. You have the ability to accomplish; you no longer have any reason to keep yourself from trying. No, you needn't pursue them all at once; start with the one most easily attained to give you the experience to tackle a harder one next.

Keep challenging yourself. Why do people climb Mount Everest? The answer is not the often-heard "because it's there." It's because each climber looks at the imposing mountain as a personal challenge, a test she/he dares to take. Find your own Mount Everests to conquer, the next always greater than the last. The more you please and satisfy yourself, the more interesting you make yourself to others, too.

Above all, trust in yourself, in your ability to develop and project those qualities that make you special. At times, you will experience some nagging doubt, a little demon that tries to get you to backtrack a bit. Go back to your mirror, repeat your "I'm terrific" speech yet another time. This time, however, when you walk away from that mirror, you will hear from within a stronger voice telling you exactly how terrific you are and you will see the reflection of your allure in the expression of everyone you meet.

About the Author

Julie Davis writes the books women want to read. Her works include both contemporary and historical novels and a wide variety of non-fiction, notably fifteen beauty, health and lifestyle titles for women of all ages. She was sixteen when she wrote her first book and nineteen when she graduated from the University of Pennsylvania and moved back home to New York to write full-time. *Allure* is her 30th book, and most personal work. She is married to Charles Goldstein, a fashion industry executive.